i

TESTIMONIALS

TO WHOM IT MAY CONCERN

RE: Dr. Rao Konduru's Publications:
Reversing Obesity
Reversing Sleep Apnea
Reversing Insomnia

Dr. Rao Konduru, PhD is a patient of mine who has suffered from chronic diabetes for most of his life; He also suffered from uncontrollable obesity, sleep apnea and chronic insomnia for the past 3 to 4 years. He has managed to reverse all of these conditions by taking non-pharmacological and science-based natural measures with great success. He has created 3 how-to user guides/books with regard to how he achieved this, and I recommend these books for anyone suffering from these conditions.

Sincerely,

Dr. Ali Ghahary, MD
Brentwood Medical Clinic
Burnaby, British Columbia, Canada

Dear Rao,
I read your book this weekend and it is an impressively comprehensive and extremely well-documented review of the broad spectrum of therapies available to treat and help relieve sleep apnea. You are to be heartily congratulated on a finely-researched and very practical work that will be accessible and useful to a wide audience of readers. I wish you every success.

Best regards,

Mr. Martin R. Hoke
President
RhinoSystems, Inc.
Brooklyn Heights, OH-44131
USA

This book "Reversing Sleep Apnea" is the true story of Dr. RK's yet another victory, this time over obstructive sleep apnea. We have read the book cover to cover. We were blown away by its extremely impressive contents, the breathtaking performance of Dr. RK and by the successful results he achieved.

obstructive sleep apnea is one of the most difficult sleep disorders that can ever be reversed by anyone in a lifetime. But Dr. RK did it in 22 months with courage, wisdom, diligence and discipline. Perhaps he is the only one in the entire world who did it to this perfection. His extensive scientific research experience and his powerful knowledge have helped him battle and combat this dangerous life challenge, and emerge a winner. This victory came along with his glorious victory over obesity, for which we all should be proud.

This book has all the information about therapies, resources and research that every sleep apnea patient, practicing doctor, nurse or technician would ever need, in a quick glance. Grab your copy sooner rather than later.

 - Prime Publishing Co.
New Westminster, British Columbia, Canada

If you are suffering from obstructive sleep apnea, this book "Reversing Sleep Apnea" ought to be your go-to guide. After living with this disorder for 22 months, Dr. RK invented a cure for his obstructive sleep apnea by identifying and removing the root cause of it. It is indeed the right way to do it.

I really appreciate the time and effort he has put into explaining the fundamentals of snoring, sleep apnea and various helpful home-based therapies with easy-to-follow and step-by-step instructions. More interestingly, he teaches us how to know if a therapy is working or not.

A must-read book for anyone with sleep apnea!

- Ms. Muriel D'Souza, Advertising Copywriter, Vancouver, British Columbia, Canada

----

++

REVIEWS

Please do not ignore reviews. Please read all reviews thoroughly.
You can learn a lot by reading through the reviews below:

++

Jade
5.0 out of 5 stars Scientific Proof Exists on Reversing Obstructive Sleep Apnea!
Reviewed in the United States on February 2, 2021
Verified Purchase

This inspirational guidebook provides us with the scientific proof that exists to reverse sleep apnea. There are scientific journal publications revealing the fact that sleep apnea can be reversed by losing weight. Whether you are obese or overweight and diagnosed with sleep apnea, you must refer to this book and I bet you will certainly get inspired and benefited!

Dr. Gary Foster, a clinical psychologist and obesity investigator, the former founder and director of the Center for Obesity Research and Education at Temple University in Philadelphia, Pennsylvania, USA where he was the Professor of Medicine, Public Health and Psychology, published several research papers confirming that the symptoms of obstructive sleep apnea and the desaturation index (defined as the number of sleep apnea events or episodes per hour) can significantly be reduced among obese people by losing at least 10% of the body weight. The more weight a sleep apnea patient loses, the more effective and successful the reversal of obstructive sleep apnea could be.

Dr. Erik Hemmingsson and Dr. Kari Johansson along with their fellow-researchers of the Karolinska Institute, Sweden published a paper in December 2009 in the British Medical Journal, concluding that weight loss can definitely help cure moderate sleep apnea and severe sleep apnea.

Dr. RK in this book "Reversing Sleep Apnea: Proof that sleep Apnea Can be Reversed By Losing Weight" provides us with the real time data of his weight loss results and the procedures he developed and adopted on how to lose weight fast and how to reverse sleep apnea by losing weight. When he lost 40 pounds of his body weight, his body mass index (BMI) was calculated to be perfectly normal. He reported that when his body resumed perfectly normal weight, his obstructive sleep apnea and other health disorders disappeared once and for all.

++

Carolyn Grigsby
5.0 out of 5 stars   well written book!
Reviewed in the United States on December 13, 2019
Reversing Sleep Apnea is the book of that kind which am reading for the very first time and this book makes me very clear about this topic.

++

+++

Anamaría Aguirre Chourio
5.0 out of 5 stars How to Fight & Reverse Obstructive Sleep Apnea!
Reviewed in the United States on March 8, 2020
Verified Purchase

After reading the very impressive books "(i) Drinking Water Guide, (ii) Permanent Diabetes Control, (iii) The Secret to Controlling Type 2 Diabetes" authored by Dr. RK, I decided to purchase and read his "Reversing Sleep Apnea" book as well. Many people with diabetes develop also sleep apnea over time. And it is known that sleep apnea disease could cause diabetes at least to some sleep apnea patients.

Reversing sleep apnea is not at all an easy task, and losing weight is extremely difficult especially when you are suffering from sleep apnea, because sleep apnea prevents weight loss. But this smart book of reversing sleep apnea shows you all those carefully planned tips, tricks and tactics on how to lose weight in those difficult circumstances, how to accomplish your weight loss goal, and ultimately how to reverse the obstructive sleep apnea.

Even if you cannot completely reverse the sleep disorder with which you have been struggling, you will be able to significantly improve your SpO2 level (percentage oxygen saturation), and the number of sleep apnea events per hour (what is known as Oxygen Desaturation Index), which must be your goal in treating sleep apnea, whether the reversal is possible or not. Improving those numbers will certainly improve your condition, and make you feel a lot better. This book teaches all about it if you have patience to read and digest the contents.

This book must be "Your 1, 2, 3 Easy Guide" as it contains the spoon-feeding instructions. It will feed you with all the fundamentals necessary in understanding the dangerous conditions such as "snoring and sleep apnea", and it will assist you in self-curing sleep apnea like a pro. Certainly and definitely, "Reversing Sleep Apnea" book overall is the extremely useful and practical guide, and therefore it is highly recommended!

+++

Radpaikr
5.0 out of 5 stars Do-It-Yourself Sleep Apnea Guide!
Reviewed in India on June 10, 2021
Verified Purchase
After I read this book, I purchased a wrist pulse oximeter on the Internet, I learned and started doing my own overnight pulse oximeter test independently at home without depending on sleep clinics in hospitals, CPAP vendors, or doctors. By monitoring and record-keeping frequently all by myself, I improved my mean SPO2 level and Desaturation Index significantly simply by losing my excess body weight. Even though I could not reverse my sleep apnea completely, I feel a lot better than ever before. I am certain that this comprehensive guide would help many sleep apnea patients. Thanks to this wonderful Sleep Apnea Guide!

+++

++

rajinder saini
5.0 out of 5 stars   This book is extremely helpful to cure my sleep apnea!
Reviewed in India on May 18, 2020
Verified Purchase

I have been living naively without taking proper care of my sleep apnea. The sleep apnea doctors and CPAP vendors never teach their patients on "how to reverse sleep apnea" but rather keep their patients hooked up to the CPAP machine for the lifetime. My doctor took overnight pulse oximetry test for me many times, and he never discussed with me about the results. I never understood those test results because I have been living naively.

After reading this book, I understood clearly what the Desaturation Index is, and what the percentage oxygen saturation (SpO2) is. As recommended in this book, I purchased the "wrist pulse oximeter for continuous monitoring" online, and started doing my own "overnight pulse oximetry test" once every few months. After doing this test overnight, early in the morning, I upload the data from my wrist pulse oximeter to my computer, and the software installed on my computer displays the test results on my computer such as Desaturation Index, Mean SpO2, Lowest SpO2, Highest SpO2. By comparing the previous test results with the current test results, I can understand my sleep apnea progress.

When I lost close to 20 pounds, my Desaturation Index decreased significantly but it is still not normal (it is not yet under 5). I still have to lose a lot more weight to lower my Desaturation Index to perfectly normal. I am now feeling now a lot better than before. Since I don't have any blockage in my throat, nose or mouth, and as I have excess body weight, I should be able to fully reverse my obstructive sleep apnea. I am now inspired to fully reverse my sleep apnea, and I will do it. Thanks to this wonderful and extremely useful book "Reversing Sleep Apnea: Proof that Sleep Apnea Can be Reversed by Losing Weight".

++

Elizabeth Wiggins
5.0 out of 5 stars   Great Book!!!
Reviewed in the United States on October 18, 2019
Format: Kindle Edition   Verified Purchase

Really, this book provides very good guidance about Reversing Sleep Apnea. I express my sincere gratitude to have this book. I learn so many new things from this book. If you have been diagnosed with obstructive sleep apnea, whether severe, moderate or mild, it is a life challenge to deal with and battle with because of the careless and unhealthy living habits you have adopted. You have been eating out way too often, not exercising enough, and have been adding pounds to your weight. Obesity is the major cause of obstructive sleep apnea. It is your responsibility to accept this challenge and take quick action against this sleep disorder you have developed. If you want to know about all these things then I think this book will be best for you. I think everyone should read this book, that's why I highly refer this book for everyone!!!

++

+++

Wellness Books
5.0 out of 5 stars   Principal Guide for Sleep Apnea Sufferers!
Reviewed in Canada on March 4, 2020
Verified Purchase
I recommend this "Reversing Sleep Apnea" book to all sleep apnea patients.

Dr. RK'S BOOKS ARE ALL MUST-READ HEALTH BOOKS: I have read his intriguing book "Drinking Water Guide". His book "Permanent Diabetes Control" is wonderful. All his health books are extremely impressive, extremely interesting, extremely useful, and directly applicable to current-day health problems that many people face today. I recommend that both medical doctors and naturopathic doctors should read these books, and benefit from the contents. All his books are science-based and practical guides. His extensive scientific research experience is clearly visible in these books.

He teaches everything so nicely step-by-step by dividing the book's contents into many headings, sub-headings and paragraphs so that a layperson can easily understand his teachings. He always convinces the reader with logic by making simple calculations that make sense. All his teachings are science-based with simple mathematics and attractive tables, showing the innovative experiments he conducted at the comfort of his home on his own body, resolving his own complex health issues with natural methods, without ever using traditional prescription drugs being prescribed by doctors. This book is no different.

I have read and enjoyed his three well-written and well-organized books "Reversing Obesity, Reversing Sleep Apnea, and Reversing Insomnia." These books are extremely useful to medical community. All contents are directly applicable to my own health problems I have been facing for years, and extremely useful. I am now using his books and am sure these books will help me controlling my weight gain, my mild sleep apnea and help cure my insomnia (sleeplessness) as well. I offer my hearty congratulations to the author Dr. RK.

+++

Steve_M
5.0 out of 5 stars Impressively Comprehensive All-In-One Sleep Apnea Guide!
Reviewed in the United States on June 13, 2021
Verified Purchase

This book is awesome, well-organized, well-written, and filled with interesting facts, anecdotes and worth-reading quotes and paragraphs. Given below is a worth-reading paragraph:

Obesity is the major cause of obstructive sleep apnea. When a person is overweight or obese, the fat cells infiltrate the neck and throat tissues so they lose firmness and are more likely to collapse on to the upper airway of the throat, thereby blocking the airway. At the same time, the neck and chin become enlarged and the airway becomes narrower. Too much weight gain also compresses the chest and makes it difficult to inhale deeply and freely. Sleep apnea statistics indicate that not only can obesity cause obstructive sleep apnea (OSA), obstructive sleep apnea (OSA) can also worsen obesity. Disrupted sleep due to apneas causes the ghrelin level to go up, and leptin level to go down. Leptin produces the feeling of satiety whereas ghrelin has the opposite effect. When this happens, low leptin levels make you eat more and as a result you gain weight. Weight gain and obstructive sleep apnea go hand in hand.

If you are diagnosed with obstructive sleep apnea as a result of severe weight gain, this book can save your life, and help you reverse your obstructive sleep apnea in a matter of months if not years. Prescribe this book to your sleep apnea doctor, and tell your doctor to read this book before he prescribes you and puts you on CPAP therapy for decades, or until the end of your life.

+++

Daniele D'Alessio
5.0 out of 5 stars Impressively Comprehensive Sleep Apnea Guide!
Reviewed in the United Kingdom on August 24, 2020
Verified Purchase

Normal SpO2 (Percentage Saturation of Oxygen in the Blood) at sea level is between 96% and 99%. Sleep apnea develops when a person's SpO2 level falls below this normal range while sleeping. For a sleep apnea patient, the blood oxygen level falls below normal due to the blockage in airway located in the throat. Whenever the SpO2 level goes down significantly during the sleep, the brain wakes the patient up so that he/she can breathe in oxygen in order make up the falling oxygen level. The occurrence of this kind of activity too many times during the night causes chronic insomnia because the brain keeps waking the patient up way too many times. Which obviously means the sleep apnea and chronic insomnia are interconnected. Most sleep apnea patients also suffer from chronic insomnia.

The CPAP therapy keeps the SpO2 level perfectly normal during the sleep as long as there are no leaks in the face mask. By means of CPAP therapy, a patient can control both sleep apnea and chronic insomnia. I have read several books on sleep apnea, but nobody explained the meaning of the CPAP and CPAP Therapy as good as this author.

CPAP means "Continuous Positive Airway Pressure," which further means that the CPAP machine helps maintain continuous, positive, very low and comfortable pressure in the airway of your throat, keeps the airway open all the time, and stops snoring whenever you sleep with it. As long as you wear the CPAP machine during the night while sleeping, the CPAP machine kills most apneas and hypopneas, and keeps your AHI (Apnea Hypopnea Index) perfectly normal. As the airway remains always open, sufficient amount of air passes into the lungs freely, and maintains normal blood oxygen levels (SpO2 = 96% to 99%) all the time during sleep. You wake up in the morning fully satisfied with your sleep and completely refreshed. You would not experience the symptoms of obstructive sleep apnea, such as tiredness with low energy, when you wake up in the morning. As you sleep all the night with perfectly normal SpO2 levels, your overall health improves. If you take appropriate steps to lose weight, your obstructive sleep apnea will be progressively healed and even reversed.

++

+++

Jack mckeever
5.0 out of 5 stars   Reversing Sleep Apnea Step-By-Step
Reviewed in the United Kingdom on March 2, 2020
Verified Purchase
This book describes sleep apnea like we can find that info nowhere else. Many people struggle to lose weight if obstructive sleep apnea disease is festering quietly in their bodies. It is known that obstructive sleep apnea prevents weight loss, and blocks weight-loss attempts. When someone has obstructive sleep apnea, the brain mistakenly thinks that the person would be starving in the near future, and causes the liver to store and hold the fat for the future use.

THIS BOOK TEACHES how to lose weight in those critical circumstances by fighting against this dangerous condition, against this sleep disorder, and against all odds. When the total calorie intake is drastically reduced, when you stop eating all those junk foods (processed foods and refined foods in restaurants, food courts, corner stores and gas bars), and when you start eating only whole foods, when you run on treadmill against all odds longer than usual, and when you exercise high self-discipline and high willpower on yourself in order to implement the above-mentioned weight-loss strategies, the stubborn fat on your stomach melts away day by day right in front of your eyes.

This book provides the real proof that when the body resumes its perfectly normal weight, the obstructive sleep apnea disappears. I am so glad and indebted that I learned the above-mentioned research-based and extremely useful strategies to reverse obstructive sleep apnea from this wonderful and resourceful book "Reversing Sleep Apnea."

+++

Rosie B.
5.0 out of 5 stars Lower Your Oxygen Desaturation Index Using This Book!
Reviewed in the United Kingdom on October 13, 2021
Verified Purchase
This book has many treatment methods to relieve and reverse obstructive sleep apnea, very beautifully explained in a very convincing way with scientific details. Doctors don't teach you how to lower your Oxygen Desaturation Index (ODI), but this is the only book that shows you everything about improving and reversing obstructive sleep apnea (OSA).

Many people with type 2 diabetes are also likely to develop sleep apnea, and the sleep apnea disease over time can lead to type 2 diabetes. I have lowered my Oxygen Desaturation Index (ODI) at least by 10 points by losing excess body weight exactly as recommended in this book. This book is packed with colossal sums of information to understand the fundamentals of sleep apnea topic, and is quite accommodating, impressive and enjoyable. I enjoyed the writer's methodology, well-researched and blended with knowledgeable information in every chapter. Everything in this book unquestionably makes sense and I found it useful in all respects. I realized that this book indeed would be helpful in every possible way to improve and reverse sleep apnea.

+++

+++

Sunil Chandel
5.0 out of 5 stars Covering A to Z of Sleep Apnea Topic!
Reviewed in India on October 10, 2021
Verified Purchase

The individual who composed this remarkable book has done a superb job indeed. I can easily imagine as my instinct tells me that the author who composed this book must be a highly educated individual who is trying to help sleep apnea victims. This book could save your life like a miracle. I will most likely refer this book to all my family members and to all my friends who have been suffering from dangerous sleep apnea disease for many years.

Energetic, dynamic and extremely helpful contents covering A to Z of sleep apnea topic are in this guide. There is a unique importance in the book that will assure you an unprecedented cure for all those who suffer from chronic sleep apnea. This guide will abolish and relieve all those underlying vicious sleep apnea symptoms in a timely fashion. Much obliged to the writer for giving the sleep apnea community such a wonderful book.

+++

Harshit srivastava
5.0 out of 5 stars Extremely Useful Sleep Apnea Guidebook!
Reviewed in India on October 12, 2021
Verified Purchase

This is an extremely useful sleep apnea guidebook for those who suffer from chronic sleep apnea. Doctors never teach the things you find in this resourceful guidebook. Doctors and CPAP vendors hook you up to a CPAP machine for lifetime, and make you a lifetime dependant patient of their practice. All they tell you is that sleep apnea cannot be reversed and so you must sleep with CPAP machine for the rest of your life, which is untrue. Many patients live with ignorance and they never realize that sleep apnea can be reversed. They even scoff and laugh if someone reversed sleep apnea.

There is scientific proof that that obstructive sleep apnea can be reversed either partly or fully. It all depends on how seriously the patient tries to lose his/her excess body weight. A patient must equip his/her mind with proper knowledge by reading this book and by mastering the concepts. One's own reading and researching efforts on how to control or completely reverse sleep apnea would guide to reverse this harmful disease. This book teaches you everything you need to reverse obstructive sleep apnea. If you have sleep apnea, this is a must-read book!

+++

++

Deanna Maio
5.0 out of 5 stars Impressively Comprehensive Sleep Apnea Book!
Reviewed in the United States on August 27, 2020
Verified Purchase

Scientists from Karolinska Institute, Sweden (a research-led medical university in Solna within the Stockholm urban area of Sweden) published a paper in Dec 2009 in the British Medical Journal, concluding and revealing the scientific fact that weight loss can definitely help cure moderate sleep apnea and severe sleep apnea.

This book "Reversing Sleep Apnea" provides the very practical proof that sleep apnea can be reversed by losing weight. The author of this book Dr. RK provided all the real-time data on how he successfully reversed his obstructive sleep apnea. He reported that his Desaturation Index dropped from 28 events/hr to 0.6 event/hour when he lost 40 pounds of his body weight, and when he lowered his body mass index (BMI) to perfectly normal.

If you have any physical obstruction or blockage in your throat, nose or mouth, it is not possible to fully reverse your sleep apnea. However, depending on how much excess body weight you have, you can always improve your Desaturation Index (number of sleep apnea events/hour) by losing weight, and feel good. If you developed obstruction sleep apnea caused due to excessive weight gain, you can fully reverse your sleep apnea and lower your Desaturation Index to normal by losing all that excess body weight. There are many scientific papers revealing this fact. This book discusses about those scientific publications.

This is the only book that has everything a sleep apnea patient needs to learn and gain concept regarding this dangerous sleep disorder. This book is very resourceful and so every sleep apnea patient should benefit from it by reading and understanding all the therapies so nicely explained. One of those therapies could suit your disorder and could free you from sleep apnea, or improve your sleep disorder. You need to try and stick to the therapy that suits your body and your sleep disorder.

++

Landon Simmons
5.0 out of 5 stars Impressive book
October 10, 2019
Format: Kindle EditionVerified Purchase
Impressive book and it provides many good points about reversing sleep apnea. The content of this book is extremely good for the beginners. I am totally impressed and I will highly recommend it to all my friends.

++

FOREWORD

PART-A

Scientists from Karolinska Institute, Sweden (a research-led medical university in Solna within the Stockholm urban area of Sweden) published a paper in Dec 2009 in the British Medical Journal, concluding and revealing the scientific fact that weight loss can definitely help cure moderate sleep apnea and severe sleep apnea.

American researchers from Obesity Research and Education, Temple University School of Medicine, Philadelphia, Pennsylvania, USA published several papers in DiabetesCare, JAMA Internal Medicine (a monthly peer-reviewed medical journal published by the American Medical Association), and in other medical journals revealing the fact that there is a strong association among the conditions obesity, type 2 diabetes and obstructive sleep apnea. Many obese people with type 2 diabetes were diagnosed with obstructive sleep apnea. Several randomized studies conducted by researchers indicated that weight loss significantly lowered the Desaturation Index (number of sleep apnea events per hour) in obese people and so it is possible to reverse obstructive sleep apnea by losing weight.

This book "Reversing Sleep Apnea authored by Dr. RK" provides the very practical proof that sleep apnea can be reversed by losing weight. Dr. RK provided all the real-time data on how he successfully reversed his obstructive sleep apnea. He reported that his Desaturation Index dropped from 28 events/hr to 0.6 event/hour when he lost 40 pounds of his body weight, and when he lowered his body mass index (BMI) to perfectly normal.

If you have any physical obstruction or blockage in your throat, nose or mouth, it is not possible to fully reverse your sleep apnea. However, depending on how much excess body weight you have, you can always improve your Desaturation Index (number of sleep apnea events/hour) and Mean SpO_2 (percentage saturation of oxygen in the blood) by losing weight. By improving the Desaturation Index and Mean SpO_2, a sleep apnea patient can feel a lot better. If you developed obstruction sleep apnea, caused due to excessive weight gain, you can fully reverse your sleep apnea and lower your Desaturation Index to perfectly normal by losing all that excess body weight. There are many scientific papers with randomized studies revealing this fact. This book discusses about those scientific publications.

This is the only book that has everything a sleep apnea patient needs to learn and gain concept regarding this dangerous sleep disorder. This book is very resourceful and so every sleep apnea patient should benefit from it by reading and understanding all the therapies so nicely explained. One of those therapies could suit your disorder and could free you from sleep apnea, or improve your sleep disorder. You need to try and stick to the therapy that suits your body and your sleep disorder.

…….. continued next page

PART-B

If you have been diagnosed with obstructive sleep apnea, whether severe, moderate or mild, it is a life challenge to deal with and battle with because of the careless and unhealthy living habits you have adopted. You have been eating out way too often, not exercising enough, and have been adding pounds to your weight. Obesity is the major cause of obstructive sleep apnea. It is your responsibility to accept the challenge and take quick action against this sleep disorder you have developed.

With determination and steadfastness, you can not only improve your condition, but also strengthen your ability to respond to your body's functionality and lead a much better life. You should always remember that knowledge is the power, so you must equip your mind with a deep understanding of sleep apnea by collecting as much information as possible, and by reading and researching a lot. Get ready to battle.

Your biggest decision is to commit to setting goals and objectives, focusing on your goal and staying focused until you fully manifest your goal. Motivation, commitment, a strong desire to succeed, self-discipline and high willpower are the essential qualities you need to implement on yourself to be successful. By awakening the giant within yourself, you can become a sleep apnea guru.

You Will Go On CPAP Therapy: CPAP means "Continuous Positive Airway Pressure," which further means that the CPAP machine pumps air into your throat, and helps maintain continuous, positive, very low and comfortable air pressure in the airway of your throat, keeps the airway open all the time, and stops snoring whenever you sleep with it.As long as you wear the CPAP machine during the night while sleeping, the CPAP machine kills most apneas and hypopneas, and keeps your AHI (Apnea Hypopnea Index) perfectly normal, under 5. As the airway remains always open, sufficient amount of air passes into the lungs freely, and maintains normal blood oxygen levels (SpO2 = 96% to 99%) all the time during sleep. You wake up in the morning fully satisfied with your sleep and completely refreshed. You would not experience the symptoms of obstructive sleep apnea, such as tiredness with low energy, when you wake up in the morning. As you sleep all the night with perfectly normal SpO2 levels, your overall health improves. If you take appropriate steps to lose weight, your obstructive sleep apnea will be progressively healed and even reversed.

You will love learning and mastering the concept of eating whole foods only and avoiding processed and refined foods. You will become an active member of a local gym, and start exercising every day. It is very likely that you will lose some weight naturally without ever using drugs or hunger suppressants prescribed by your doctor. Even some 10 to 20 pounds of weight loss would have a significant impact on your sleep apnea progress. The number of sleep apnea events per hour during your sleep would significantly decline, switching you from severe to moderate or from moderate to mild sleep apnea, and allowing you to feel a lot better than you have ever felt since your diagnosis.

However a substantial weight loss that lowers your Body Mass Index (BMI) to perfectly normal (18.5 to 24.9 Kg/m ^{2}) would completely wipe out sleep apnea from your body. This is a proven fact, believe it or not. You will be amazed to witness your own breathtaking performance and live with a joyous feeling as your "overnight pulse oximetry test" would reveal that your sleep apnea has just been reversed, and that you are free. You would declare yourself a proud winner in the battle against sleep apnea. Many surrounding people would be intimidated, become envious and a few even surprised.

You would no longer be sleeping with the CPAP machine. You could pack your CPAP machine and accessories in a bag and leave it in your closet or even sell it off on Craigslist. This is what exactly happened to Dr. RK who wrote the book "Reversing Sleep Apnea."

-- Prime Publishing Co.

COPYRIGHT

Copyright © 2018-2026 and Beyond by the Author .
All rights reserved under International and Pan-American Copyright laws.
This book "Reversing Sleep Apnea" is revised and rewritten in 2026.

Dr. Rao Konduru's Publications	
1. Permanent Diabetes Control	www.mydiabetescontrol.com
2. The Secret to Controlling Type 2 Diabetes	www.mydiabetescontrol.com
3. Reversing Obesity	www.reversingsleepapnea.com/ebook2.html
4. Reversing Sleep Apnea	www.reversingsleepapnea.com
5. Reversing Insomnia	www.reversinginsomnia.com
6. Drinking Water Guide	www.drinkingwaterguide.com

The paperbacks (softcover books) and Kindle eBooks are available for purchase on Amazon.com for US residents, and on Amazon.ca for Canadian residents.

TABLE OF CONTENTS

CHAPTER 1 SLEEP APNEA STATISTICS

Nearly 1 Billion People Worldwide Have Sleep Apnea!

TABLE OF CONTENTS

CHAPTER 1   SLEEP APNEA STATISTICS

1. Statistics Reported By NCBI, ResMed and Others [1, 2, 3]
Nearly 1 Billion People Worldwide Have Sleep Apnea

◦Researchers most recently analyzed prevalence studies from 16 countries, together with data from the World Health Organization and United Nations World Population Prospects, and concluded that "Nearly 1 Billion People Worldwide Have Sleep Apnea." The previous estimation of 100 million by World Health Organization in 2007 was proved to be false. The current analyses included only people aged 30 to 69 years, which obviously means that the real number could be a lot more than 1 billion people.

◦China had the highest prevalence of obstructive sleep apnea (OSA), followed by the United States, Brazil and India. Pakistan, Russia, Nigeria, Germany, France and Japan were also in the top 10 list. These numbers reflected the population size of each country.

2. Star Wars Actress "Carrie Fisher" Died from Sleep Apnea in 2017 [4, 5]

◦The American Academy of Sleep Medicine (AASM) has issued a warning emphasizing how dangerous sleep apnea is after confirming the cause of death of the 60-year old Star Wars actress Carrie Fisher, who died on December 27, 2017, as "severe sleep apnea."
The doctors determined that the actress Carrie Fisher died after suffering from "**Untreated Obstructive Severe Sleep Apnea,**" for a long time.

◦The word apnea means "breathing stopped." When a person suffers from obstructive sleep apnea, the airway in the throat is either partly or fully obstructed or blocked several times in an ongoing manner throughout the night, thereby lowering the oxygen concentration in the blood to below normal. This sleep disturbance contributes itself to various health consequences, including but not limited to excessive daytime sleepiness, tiredness, fatigue, heavy snoring, and non-refreshing sleep. Obstructive sleep apnea, when left untreated, increases the risk of atherosclerotic heart disease (coronary artery disease), heart attack, heart failure, high blood pressure, type 2 diabetes, stroke, depression, and other ailments.

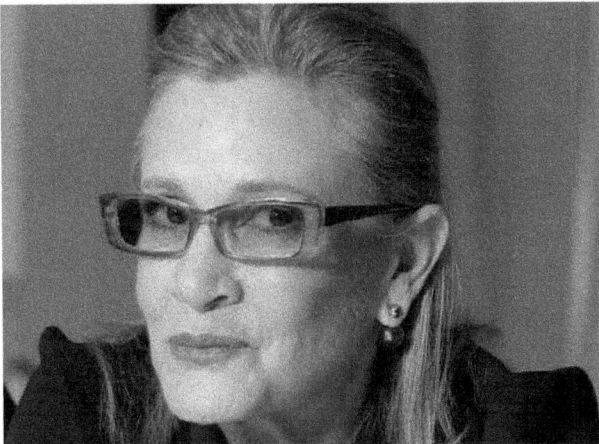

Star Wars Actress "Carrie Fisher" died from Untreated Obstructive Sleep Apnea (OSA).

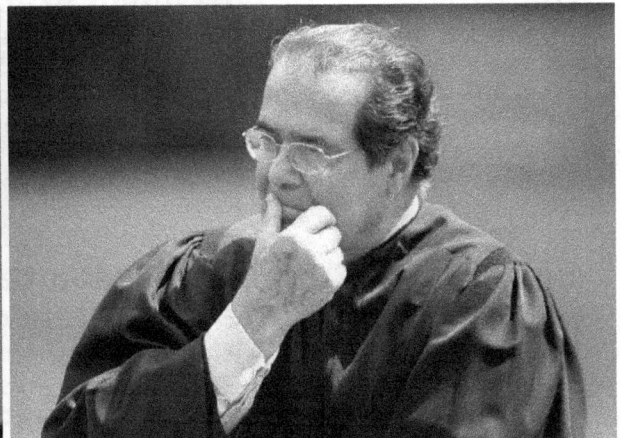

Supreme Court Justice "Honourable Antonin Scalia" died in his sleep when he forgot to hook himself up to his CPAP machine and slept without CPAP.

3. Supreme Court Justice "Antonin Scalia" Died in His Sleep in 2016 [6, 7]
At the age of 79 on Feb 13, 2016, supreme court justice "Honourable Antonin Scalia" died in his sleep when he forgot to hook himself up to his CPAP machine and slept. Doctors figured out that justice Antonin Scalia has been living with numerous serious health problems such as heart disease, type 2 diabetes and high blood pressure for years as a consequence of obstructive sleep apnea. Justice Antonin Scalia is one of an estimated 22 million Americans who have sleep apnea.

⦁ There are very many other actors, athletes and celebrities, around the world, living with and battling sleep apnea. Millions of men and women with sleep apnea are unaware of the aforementioned serious risk factors, and naively remain undiagnosed and untreated for a long time. Many people don't realize that with an early diagnosis and appropriate treatment, the risk factors and complications of sleep apnea can be minimized and even reversed.

Obstructive sleep apnea is a common but serious sleep disorder that repeatedly causes a person to stop breathing during the sleep, thereby lowering the oxygen saturation in the blood (SpO2 level) significantly. The stress that sleep apnea causes on heart and brain of a person can be so severe and harmful that long-term health consequences could be fatal, unbearable and dangerous, and could eventually lead to death.

4. Statistics Reported By ResMed [8]
The following statistics were reported by a CPAP manufacturing company ResMed:
- ⦁ Approximately 42 million American adults have sleep disordered breathing (SDB).
- ⦁ 1 in 5 adults has mild obstructive sleep apnea (OSA).
- ⦁ 1 in 15 has moderate to severe OSA.
- ⦁ 9% of middle-aged women and 25% of middle-aged men suffer from OSA.
- ⦁ Prevalence similar to asthma (20 million) and diabetes (23.6 million) of US population.
- ⦁ 75% of severe SDB cases remain undiagnosed.

5. Statistics Reported By Men's Health [9]
⦁ Around 50 to 70 million Americans get poor or insufficient sleep. [8] An estimated 4 percent to 6 percent of American men suffer from sleep apnea, and most of them deny and don't even realize how dangerous the sleep apnea is.

6. The University of Wisconsin Statistical Survey [10]
⦁ The University of Wisconsin, Madison statistical survey revealed the fact that the death rate among sleep apnea sufferers tripled in 18 years. In 1989, Dr. Terry Young, an epidemiologist (a person who studies diseases within populations of people) conducted a sleep apnea study in the University of Wisconsin, Madison. Around 1522 Wisconsin state employees participated and underwent the overnight sleep apnea testing called "polysomnogram." From this study, the researcher Dr. Terry Young found that 63 people (about 4% of the group) had severe sleep apnea, 20% had moderate or mild sleep apnea, and 76% had no sleep apnea.

7. Sleep Apnea Sufferers Caused Car Crashes [11]
Sleep Apnea Sufferers Developed Diabetes &
Pregnant Women With Sleep Apnea Developed Gestational Diabetes
⦁ Sleep apnea is linked to car crashes, diabetes, heart disease and even pregnancy complications in women. Dr. Alan Mulgrew, MD and his colleagues at the University of British Columbia, Vancouver, Canada compared the records of motor vehicle accidents of 800 patients who had sleep apnea with the records of another 800 patients who did not suffer from sleep apnea. Their study suggested that people with sleep apnea are five times more likely to have car crashes than those without sleep apnea.

● Another team of researchers, Bortos and his colleagues at Yale University, compared the health records of 600 patients who had sleep apnea with the health records of another 600 patients who did not suffer from sleep apnea. Their study suggested that people with sleep apnea are 2.5 times more likely to develop diabetes. Sleep apnea symptoms cause stress on the insulin-making beta cells of the pancreas, they thereby produce less insulin than required, resulting in the disease called "diabetes."

● Dr. Neomi Shah, MD and other researchers of Yale University examined the health records of 1123 patients who had sleep apnea. 500 of these patients had moderate or mild sleep apnea. It was believed that these patients could suffer a heart attack if they continued to live with the sleep apnea for another 4 to 5 years without treatment. If their sleep apnea would be appropriately treated, the researchers believed that the risk of a heart attack could be minimized.

● Dr. Hatim Youssef, DO in the University of Medicine & Dentistry of New Jersey-Robert Wood Johnson Medical School conducted some research on pregnant women and concluded that the pregnant women who gain too much weight with Body Mass Index (BMI) over 35 in the third trimester, tend to live with sleep apnea. The researchers analyzed the 2003 medical records of 4 million U.S. women who delivered babies. They found that 452 of these 4 million women had sleep apnea. These 454 women with sleep apnea were twice likely than other women to have gestational diabetes and four times more likely to have high blood pressure.

8. A Lot of Women Also Have Sleep Apnea, Not Just Men [12]
● More than 40,000 deaths occur each year from Motor Vehicle Accidents in the USA, and it is estimated that 15-20% of crashes are related to drowsy driving and sleep apnea.

● American Academy of Sleep Medicine revealed that untreated obstructive sleep apnea is associated with a higher risks of stroke and heart attack, and can increase the risk for work-related accidents and driving accidents.

● Dr. Richard Leung, St. Michael's Hospital Sleep Lab in Toronto declared the following statement: "Men who are overweight probably have the most severe sleep apnea, but that doesn't mean women and other groups can't have it."

● Franklin and the other Swedish researchers selected 400 women aged 20 to 70 from a random sample of 10,000 women, and asked them to participate in an overnight sleep study. Their study found that 50% of them were diagnosed with sleep apnea. About 14% of those 400 women were found to be living with severe sleep apnea. The study was funded by grants from the Swedish Heart-Lung Foundation.

9. Archives of Public Health Agency of Canada & Statistics Canada [13]
In 2009, the Public Health Agency of Canada (PHAC), after conducting a research in conjunction with Statistics Canada, published the following results:

● 860,000 Canadians were told by a health professional that they have sleep apnea.
● Twice as many men as women reported that they had sleep apnea.
● 25% of adults with sleep apnea rated their general health as fair or poor compared to 11% in the general population.
● 89% of adults with sleep apnea were overweight or obese, linking obesity to sleep apnea, based on self-reported height and weight.
● Patients with sleep apnea were 2.5 times more likely to report having diabetes.

• Patients with sleep apnea were 1.8 times more likely to report hypertension.
• Patients with sleep apnea were 2.2 times more likely to report heart disease.
• Patients with sleep apnea were 2.2 times more likely to report a mood disorder such as depression, bipolar disorder, mania or dysthymia.

10. Statistical Survey From 9523 Canadians [14]

The Public Health Agency of Canada funded the 2009 **Sleep Apnea Rapid Response Questionnaire** in the Canadian population. The survey, conducted by Statistics Canada as part of the Canadian Community Health Survey, interviewed a nationally representative sample of 9,523 Canadians ages 12 years and older. They came up with the following conclusions:

• An estimated 858,900 Canadian adults were told by a health care professional that they have sleep apnea.
• The prevalence of self-reported sleep apnea was 3% among adults ages 18 years and older; this rose to 5% in individuals 45 years and older.
• 3 out of 4 Canadians reporting sleep apnea (75%) were 45 years and older.
• The prevalence of self-reported sleep apnea in adult men was twice when compared to women.
• 25% of adults reporting sleep apnea rated their general health as fair or poor compared to 11% in the general population.
• Over 1 in 4 Canadian adults (26%) was at high risk for having obstructive sleep apnea.
• 73% of adults at high risk for obstructive sleep apnea were men, and 76% were over the age of 50 years.
• 12% of adults at high risk of obstructive sleep apnea were obese with a BMI greater than 35 kg/m^2.
• Many Canadians were diagnosed with sleep apnea without the benefit of sleep laboratory testing such as polysomnography. Many Canadians did the home-based self-testing by using overnight pulse oximetry at home.

11. Scientific Study: Sleep Apnea Linked to Cancer [15]

• A new animal study led by Dr. Antoni Vilaseca and other researchers from the Hospital Clinic of Barcelona of Spain presented a scientific research article at the European Association of Urology (EAU) Congress in Munich, Germany. The researchers suggested that there is a link between the sleep disorder and cancer. Researchers used 24 mice that had kidney tumors for their study. 12 of the mice were in an experimental group and the other 12 mice served as a control. After the 12 experimental mice exposed to varying oxygen levels to mimic the sleep disorder such as hypoxia (a condition in which the blood oxygen levels fall too low), researchers noticed an increased amount of vascular progenitor and endothelial cells within the kidney tumors. They interpreted that the so-called sleep disorder hypoxia could increase the size of the tumors by allowing more oxygen along with the nutrients to penetrate into the blood vessels of the tumors. The researcher Dr. Antoni Vilaseca concluded from their animal study that the patients who suffer from obstructive sleep apnea may also experience hypoxia at night, and hypoxia increases the risk of cancer by allowing the size of the cancer tumors to grow.

• Dr. Arnulf Stenzl, the chair of the EAU Congress Committee then spoke that the healthy lifestyle changes such as "not smoking" are important to those who were diagnosed with sleep apnea or hypoxia and also spoke about the association of sleep apnea or hypoxia with other health risks such as high blood pressure, stroke and depression.

12. The University of California Statistical Survey [16]

The University of California at San Diego campus studied by examining the health records of 54 African Americans and 346 Caucasians for the presence of sleep apnea.
The study revealed the following facts:

 17% of African American subjects had obstructive sleep apnea present, compared to 8% of the Caucasian subjects. This denotes a hypothesis that African Americans stand an increased risk of obstructive sleep apnea.
 The National Highway Traffic Safety Administration has stated that drowsy driving is responsible for, at the very least, 100,000 car accidents, 40,000 injuries, and 1,550 deaths per year.
 More than 263,000 children per year undergo tonsillectomies. Most of these operations are performed due to the presence of sleep apnea in the children that is caused by the tonsils obstructing their airway.
 A spouse of a person with untreated obstructive sleep apnea can lose up to an hour per night of sleep. This was discovered when a study was conducted that measured the effects of CPAP treatment in helping the spouse to sleep.
 People that have an untreated case of sleep apnea face a risk of stroke that is four times as likely as those who are not afflicted. Untreated sleep apnea sufferers are also three times as likely to have heart disease.
 On the average night's sleep, an obstructive sleep apnea sufferer may experience 60 apneas per hour. This accounts for an average of 400 apneas per night!
 Almost half of all hospital patients who have hypertension are also afflicted with sleep apnea. Conversely, around half of all sleep apnea sufferers face a diagnosis of hypertension.
 According to the National Commission on Sleep Disorders Research, approximately 38,000 deaths occur per year related to cardiovascular problems that in one way or another are connected to sleep apnea. These problems include high blood pressure and stroke.
 An estimated 6 million Americans suffer from sleep apnea. Unfortunately a great many people (about 500,000 people) do not even realize that they suffer from sleep apnea.

13. Statistics Reported By BergerHenry ENT Medical Center [17]

BergerHenry ENT Center, East Norriton, PA 19401, USA reported the most recent statistics of sleep apnea as follows:
 When left untreated, sleep apnea can cause high blood pressure and other cardiovascular disease, weight gain, memory problems, impotency and headaches. Untreated sleep apnea may also cause job impairment and vehicle accidents.
 If you have sleep apnea, you tend to be more sleepy and lack concentration. As a result, your chances of being in a car accident increase and you are 6x more likely to die in a car accident. People who drive sleepy are responsible for 100,000 car accidents, 40,000 injuries, and 1,550 deaths annually in USA alone.
 Over a quarter of a million children have tonsillectomies each year and most undergo these operations because their tonsils cause an obstruction of the airway which, in turn, cause sleep apnea.

14. 5 Surprising Facts About Sleep Apnea [18]
THE FOLLOWING ARE 5 SURPRISING FACTS ABOUT SLEEP APNEA:

(i) Many people who have sleep apnea don't know about it as their doctors do not understand their symptoms and do not diagnose them properly.
(ii) Sleep apnea happens to not just overweight men who snore, but also overweight women.
(iii) Sleep apnea may seem like depression, fatigue or something else. So don't get confused. Get it diagnosed properly.

(iv) Sleep apnea and obesity develop simultaneously by influencing one another, and may lead to very serious complications such as diabetes, heart disease, heart attack & stroke.
(v) You can do something about sleep apnea to escape: healthy lifestyle changes such as no smoking, no alcohol consumption, losing weight, sleeping on the sides but not on the back, treating insomnia, practicing yoga for a good night sleep, and using the CPAP therapy or PAP therapy or a mouthpiece if lifestyle changes don't work.

15. Statistics From Randomized Research Studies [19]

● From randomized research studies, it was estimated that 24% of men and 9% of women between 30 and 60 years old have obstructive sleep apnea (OSA).
● Approximately 9% of men and 4% of women have either moderate or severe obstructive sleep apnea (OSA). And 70% to 80% of these people do not get tested, and as a result remain undiagnosed.
● A randomized 8-year study of 282 patients showed that the AHI (Apnea Hypopnea Index) rapidly increases in overweight and obese people if sleep apnea is left untreated.

16. Mortality Risk Doubled Among People with Sleep Apnea [20, 21]

● Several randomized research studies revealed that sleep apnea may double the risk of sudden death, and has associations with an increased risk of sudden and cardiovascular-related deaths.

● The quantitative analysis included a combined total of over 42,000 individuals across the world. The meta-analysis showed that individuals with obstructive sleep apnea were approximately twice as likely to experience sudden death than those who did not have sleep apnea. The study also identified that obstructive sleep apnea resulted in a nearly twofold risk of cardiovascular death that increased with age.

● A randomized research study among 1,522 participants in an ongoing Wisconsin Sleep Cohort Study, which was established in 1988, reported the following results: Severe sleep apnea was associated with increased mortality risk. About 42 percent of deaths in people with severe sleep apnea were attributed to cardiovascular disease or stroke, compared with 26 percent of deaths in people without sleep apnea.

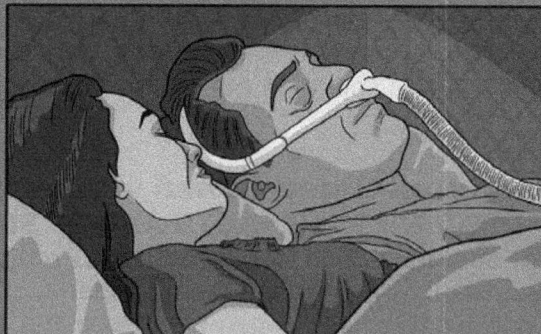

CHAPTER 1   SLEEP APNEA STATISTICS

REFERENCES

1. Nearly 1 Billion People Worldwide Have Sleep Apnea, International Sleep Experts Estimate, Posted by ResMed, Posted on May 21, 2018.
https://investor.resmed.com/investor-relations/events-and-presentations/press-releases/press-release-details/2018/Nearly-1-Billion-People-Worldwide-Have-Sleep-Apnea-International-Sleep-Experts-Estimate/default.aspx

2. OSA may affect nearly 1 billion adults worldwide by Healio, Posted on July 29, 2019.
https://www.healio.com/news/pulmonology/20190729/osa-may-affect-nearly-1-billion-adults-worldwide

3. Estimation of the global prevalence and burden of obstructive sleep apnoea: a literature-based analysis, Authoors: Adam V Benjafield, Najib T Ayas, Peter R Eastwood, Raphael Heinzer, Mary S M Ip, Mary J Morrell, Carlos M Nunez, Sanjay R Patel, Thomas Penzel, Jean-Louis D Pépin, Paul E Peppard, Sanjeev Sinha, Sergio Tufik, Kate Valentine, and Atul Malhotra, Published by NCBI (National Center for Biotechnology Information).
https://www.ncbi.nlm.nih.gov/pmc/articles/PMC7007763/

4. Death of Carrie Fisher is a warning about sleep apnea by Corinne Lederhouse, Posted on Jun 20, 2017.
http://sleepeducation.org/news/2017/06/20/death-of-Carrie-Fisher-is-a-warning-about-sleep-apnea

5. Yes You Can Die From Sleep Apnea as Carrie Fisher Did by Sleepapnea.org, Posted on June 21, 2017.
https://www.sleepapnea.org/carrie-fisher-yes-you-can-die-from-sleep-apnea/

6. Did sleep apnea contribute to Justice Scalia's death? His unplugged breathing machine raises that question by Ariana Eunjung Cha, Staff writer, Posted on Feb 24, 2016.
https://www.washingtonpost.com/news/to-your-health/wp/2016/02/24/scalia-may-have-forgotten-to-hook-himself-up-to-sleep-apnea-machine-why-that-can-be-dangerous/

7. Questions raised by Justice Scalia's unplugged breathing machine by Ariana Eunjung Cha, The Washington Post, Originally Published on February 24, 2016.
https://www.seattletimes.com/nation-world/questions-raised-by-justice-scalias-unplugged-breathing-machine/

8. Sleep Apnea Facts and Figures by ResMed, PDF File.
http://www.resmed.com/us/dam/documents/products/dental/Narval-CC/facts-and-figures/1015527r3_narval-cc-mrd_facts-and-figures_amer_eng.pdf

9. How Sleep Apnea Could be Killing You:
An estimated 4% to 6% of Americans suffer from Sleep Apnea by Jim Thornton, Photography By Thinkstock March 3, 2015.
http://www.menshealth.com/health/sleep-apnea-could-be-killing-you

10. Death Rate Triples for Sleep Apnea Sufferers, Posted by the University of Wisconsin Health Organization.
https://bittnerdentalclinic.com/death-rate-triples-sleep-apnea-sufferers/

11. Sleep Apnea Death Risks: Sleep Apnea Linked to Car Wrecks, Diabetes, Heart Attack, Pregnancy Woes, by Salynn Boyles, WebMD, May 22, 2007.
http://www.webmd.com/sleep-disorders/sleep-apnea/news/20070522/sleep-apnea-death-risks?src=rsf_full-1836_pub_none_rltd#1

12. How Many People Die of Sleep Apnea Every Year?
Is there any way to determine sleep apnea or sleep apnea related deaths in a year?
http://www.quora.com/How-many-people-die-each-year-from-sleep-apnea

13. Sleep Apnea Linked to Men also Common in Women; Snoring and Restless Sleep Tied to Obesity, High Blood Pressure, Posted by: CBC News, Aug 15, 2012.
http://www.cbc.ca/news/health/sleep-apnea-linked-to-men-also-common-in-women-1.1232346

14. What is the Impact of Sleep Apnea on Canadians? Fast Facts from the 2009 Canadian Community Health Survey (Public Health Agency of Canada) - Sleep Apnea Rapid Response
http://www.phac-aspc.gc.ca/cd-mc/sleepapnea-apneesommeil/ff-rr-2009-eng.php
http://www.phac-aspc.gc.ca/cd-mc/sleepapnea-apneesommeil/pdf/sleep-apnea.pdf

15. Common Side Effect Of Sleep Apnea, Hypoxia, May Be Associated With Worse Cancer Outcomes; 50 to 70 million Americans get poor or insufficient sleep, by Jaleesa Baulkman, Mar 12, 2016.
http://www.medicaldaily.com/sleep-apnea-hypoxia-cancer-outcomes-377689

16. Sleep Apnea Statistics by SleepDisordersGuide.com.
http://www.sleepdisordersguide.com/article/sleep-disorders/sleep-apnea-statistics-the-statistics-of-sleep-apnea

17. Sleep Apnea Statistics and Facts (2016) by BergerHenry ENT Medical Center, East Norriton, PA 19401, USA.
http://www.bergerhenryent.com/sleep-apnea-statistics-2016/

18. 5 Surprising Facts About Sleep Apnea by DeJesus Dental Group, Posted on Sept 21, 2016.
https://dejesusdental.com/blog/general-dentistry/5-surprising-facts-about-sleep-apnea/

19. Obstructive Sleep Apnea: Symptoms, Causes, Treatments and Natural Remedies by an Unknown Author, Sleep-Apnea-Guide.com, 2020.
https://www.sleep-apnea-guide.com/obstructive-sleep-apnea.html

20. Sleep apnea may almost double the risk of sudden death, Written by Leigh Ann Green, Fact checked by Rita Ponce, Ph.D., Medical News Today.
https://www.medicalnewstoday.com/articles/sleep-apnea-may-almost-double-the-risk-of-sudden-death

21. Study shows that people with sleep apnea have a high risk of death, American Academy of Sleep Medicine
https://aasm.org/study-shows-that-people-with-sleep-apnea-have-a-high-risk-of-death/

CHAPTER 2   SNORING AND SLEEP APNEA

TABLE OF CONTENTS

CHAPTER 2   SNORING AND SLEEP APNEA

SNORING EXPLAINED [1, 2, 3, 4]

Not all people who snore have sleep apnea, but almost all sleep apnea patients do snore. Snoring affects all people including adults and children. An estimated 10% to 12% of children snore. Habitual snoring affects 24% of adult women and 40% of adult men. The likelihood of snoring increases by unhealthy lifestyles such as the smoking, alcohol, sedatives and muscle relaxants if consumed a few hours before going to bed.

CAUSES OF SNORING: Snoring occurs when the flow of inhaled air through the mouth and/or the nose is physically obstructed. The obstruction of the airflow through the nose and/or the mouth is caused due to several factors such as:
a. Obstructed nasal airway,
b. Poor muscle tone in the throat and tongue,
c. Bulky throat tissue,
d. Long soft palate and/or uvula,
e. Large tonsils,
f. Unusually shaped or small mouth.

HOW SNORING OCCURS? When you breathe, air is forced into the airway through your nose, mouth and throat. If the airway in your throat is restricted, several tissues such as the soft palate (the back of the roof of the mouth), uvula, tonsils, adenoids and tongue vibrate against each other, emitting the iconic, rather hoarse, harsh, rattling or choking sound, called snoring. In other words, snoring occurs when the upper airway is partially blocked. It was also determined that snoring occurs only during the Non-REM sleep stage, meaning that it is impossible to dream while you are snoring, as dreaming occurs during REM stage of sleep.

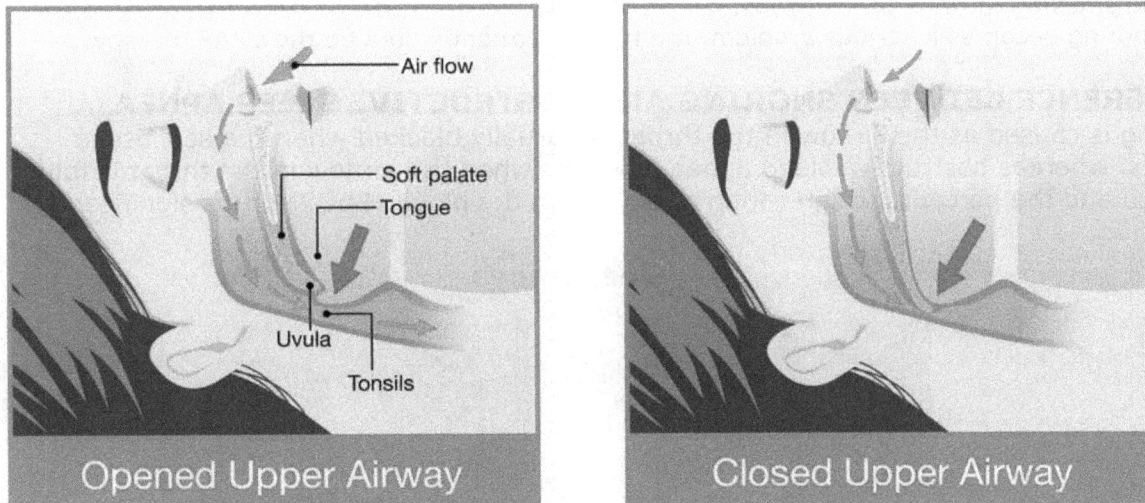

Figure 2.1 Snoring diagram (upper airway opened & upper airway partially closed).

As shown in the figure below, the soft palate is the muscles structure at the back of the roof of the mouth. The uvula is a small, finger-shaped piece of tissue that hangs down from the soft palate in the back of the throat. Tonsils are balls of tissue in the throat. Tonsils play a small role in helping your body defend against and recover from the illnesses from which you suffer. The tongue helps you talk, chew and swallow.

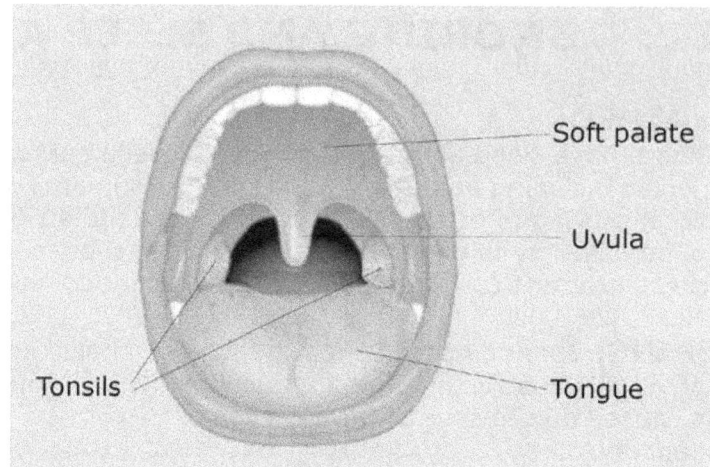

Figure 2.2 The soft palate, uvula, tonsils and tongue vibrate together, emitting snoring.

TREATMENT OF SNORING

Most people who live alone, realize themselves that they snore. Else a mate or a family member gets disturbed and informs you that you snore. There are many natural methods available to treat snoring at the comfort of your home, as described below:

a. Snoring can be completely stopped by sleeping on the side instead of on the back.

b. Snoring can be minimized or completely stopped by using some nasal strips or nasal sprays to open the obstruction in the nose.

c. Snoring can be minimized or completely stopped by wearing an appropriate vestibular guard (a kind of mouth guard), chin strap or a mouthpiece that keeps your jaw and tongue forward so that there won't be any obstruction in the airway, and airflow becomes normal when inhaling and exhaling.

d. Snoring can be minimized or completely stopped by implementing lifestyle changes such as quitting smoking, alcohol or sedatives.

e. If snoring becomes a serious problem, the best treatment would be the CPAP therapy.

DIFFERENCE BETWEEN SNORING AND OBSTRUCTIVE SLEEP APNEA

Snoring is caused as the airflow in the throat is partially blocked when the soft tissue relaxes, whereas obstructive sleep apnea develops when the airflow in the throat is fully blocked and the percentage saturation of oxygen in the blood (SpO2) drops significantly.

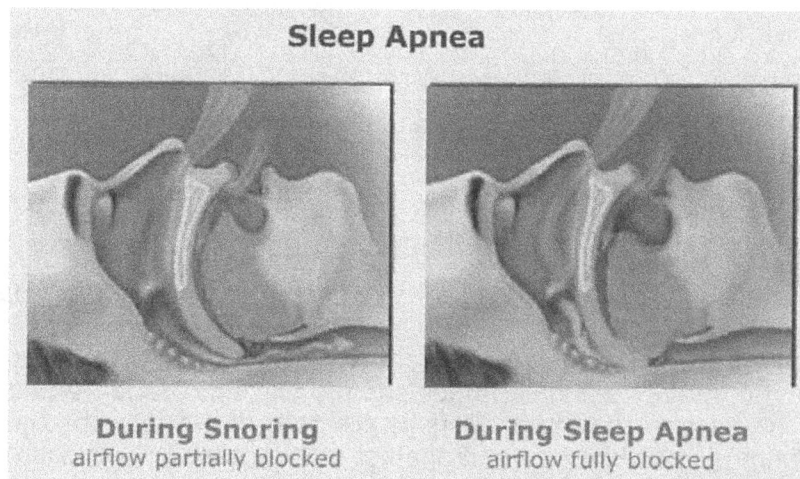

Figure 2.3 Difference between snoring and sleep apnea.

SLEEP APNEA EXPLAINED [5, 6, 7]

Obstructive sleep apnea develops due to the airway blockage in your throat, usually when the soft tissue in the rear of the throat relaxes too much and collapses during sleep. When the muscles relax, your airway narrows or closes as you breathe in, interrupting the breathing process for 10 seconds or longer, thereby lowering the blood oxygen level (SpO2 level drops).

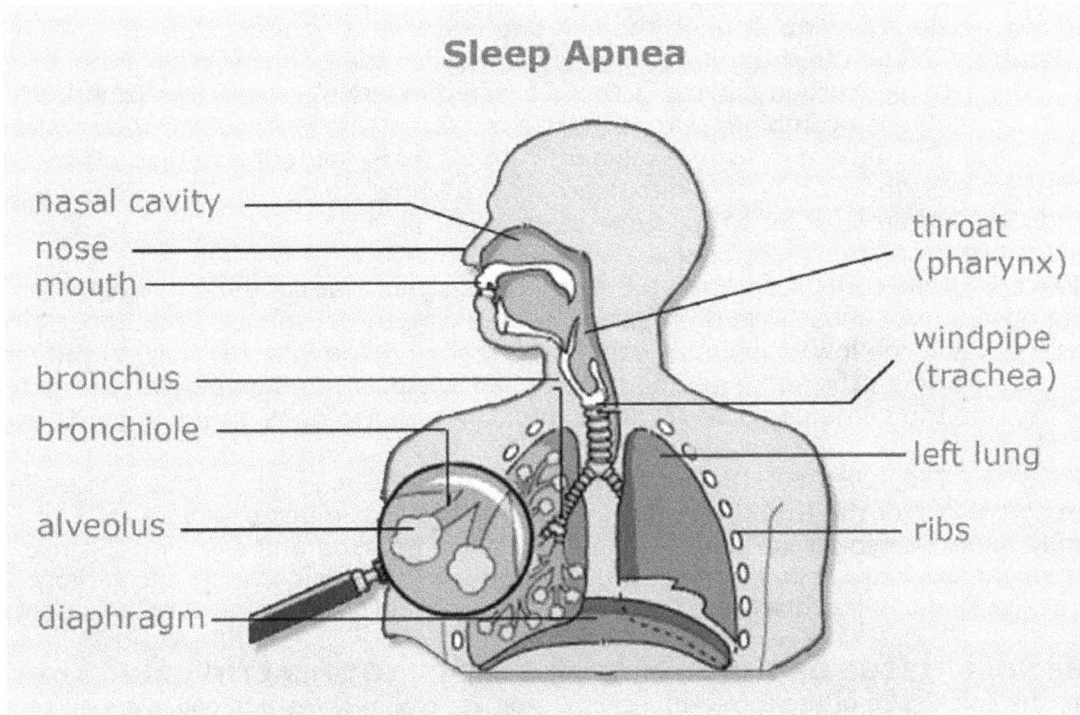

Figure 2.4 Obstructive sleep apnea picture-I.

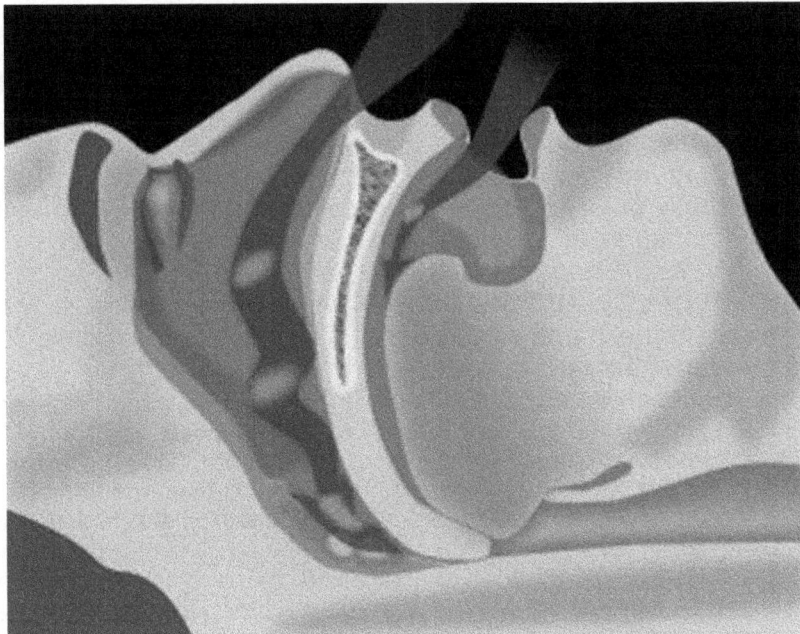

Figure 2.5 Obstructive sleep apnea picture-II (The airway in the throat is blocked).

THE BREATHING PROCESS: Humans breathe in and breathe out air through the nose and/or mouth in order to take in oxygen for their survival. Air in the atmosphere before it is inhaled contains 21% oxygen, 79% nitrogen and 0.04% carbon dioxide (CO_2). When they exhale, the air composition changes. The exhaled air contains only 16% oxygen, 79% nitrogen (nitrogen is an inert component and the human body does not consume nitrogen so its composition is unchanged), 4 to 5% carbon dioxide (CO_2) and some water vapor. Red blood cells traveling through the veins to and from the lungs consume oxygen from air, distribute oxygen to the trillions of body cells, and send out the remaining air along with the waste gas carbon dioxide (CO_2). Carbon dioxide is a waste gas produced when carbon from glucose combines with oxygen associated with energy-making processes in the body's cells. So humans consume oxygen from air by inhaling it and give off carbon dioxide (CO_2) by exhaling it. This continuous process, 24 hours a day and 7 days a week, of inhaling and exhaling air in order to consume oxygen is called "the Breathing."

THE AIRWAY IN THE THROAT: When a person inhales, air that contains oxygen flows through the nose and/or mouth via the upper airway of the throat muscle (the upper airway is called pharynx and the lower airway is called trachea/windpipe in the throat) and then into the lungs. And when the same person exhales, air with carbon dioxide (CO_2) from the lungs flows out via the same upper airway and then through the nose and/or mouth.

WHEN THE SOFT TISSUE OF THE THROAT MUSCLE IS HEALTHY: When a person falls asleep, the soft tissue of the throat muscle, <u>if healthy</u>, allows the upper airway to automatically remain open all the time during sleep while inhaling and exhaling. So the person with healthy soft tissue in the throat muscle sleeps well without snoring and without experiencing any kind of sleep disorder. The blood oxygen level (SpO2) always remains normal.

WHEN THE SOFT TISSUE OF THE THROAT MUSCLE IS NOT HEALTHY: When a person falls asleep, the soft tissue of the throat muscles, <u>if not healthy</u>, relaxes and collapses on to the upper airway of the throat, blocks it, and snoring occurs while inhaling and exhaling as shown by the blue arrow in the picture. As a result, the blood oxygen level (SpO2) falls below normal.

SLEEPING ON THE SIDES IS BETTER THAN SLEEPING ON THE BACK: That is why if you sleep on your back, the throat muscle is more prone to relax, collapse and block the airway. If you develop the habit of sleeping on your sides, as is strongly advised, you can minimize this problem of airway blockage. If this problem of airway blockage in your throat persists while you breathe in, you repeatedly suffocate yourself throughout the night, snoring worsens, and eventually obstructive sleep apnea (OSA) develops. You would then feel the symptoms of sleep apnea as listed below.

OBESE & OVERWEIGHT PEOPLE HAVE SLEEP APNEA: When a person is overweight or obese, the fat cells infiltrate the neck and throat tissues so they lose firmness and are more likely to collapse on to the upper airway of the throat, thereby blocking the airway. At the same time, the neck and chin become enlarged and the airway becomes narrower. Too much weight gain also compresses the chest and makes it difficult to inhale deeply and freely. Sleep apnea statistics indicate that not only can obesity cause obstructive sleep apnea (OSA), obstructive sleep apnea (OSA) can also worsen obesity. Disrupted sleep due to apneas causes the ghrelin level to go up, and leptin level to go down. Leptin produces the feeling of satiety whereas ghrelin has the opposite effect. When this happens, low leptin levels make you eat more and as a result you gain weight.

SLIM PEOPLE ALSO HAVE SLEEP APNEA: The obstructive sleep apnea (OSA) can also occur in slim people. The reason in this case could be due to chronic nasal congestion, enlarged or elongated tonsils and adenoids, oversized uvula, oversized tongue, or a small and undersized jaw.

TYPES OF SLEEP APNEA [8, 9, 10]

Table 2.1 Types of sleep apnea.

There are Three to Four Types of Sleep Apnea	
1. Obstructive Sleep Apnea	OBSTRUCTIVE SLEEP APNEA (OSA) IS THE MOST COMMON TYPE. In the obstructive sleep apnea (OSA), as the name suggests, the airway in the throat is partly or fully obstructed thereby blocking the passage of air into the lungs. The obstruction arises due to one or more of the following causes: (i) When obese or overweight people fall asleep, the soft tissue in the throat muscle relaxes, collapses and blocks the airway (windpipe) in the throat (ii) Chronic nasal congestion (iii) Enlarged or elongated tonsils (iv) An oversized uvula (v) An oversized tongue (vi) A small and undersized jaw (short mandible) (vii) A thick or short neck (viii) Smoking or alcohol consumption (ix) The side effects of some medication If OSA develops, the blood oxygen levels fall below normal many times during the night, causing heavy snoring and disruptive sleep episodes. In most cases, this sleep disorder can be treated with the CPAP therapy. For slim people and mouth-breathers, the CPAP machine may not work. They need a mouthpiece or supplemental oxygen.
2. Central Sleep Apnea	In central sleep apnea (CSA), the brain fails to function appropriately in order to promote normal breathing patterns. So after falling asleep the person is unable to inhale and exhale like a normal person does, even though the airway in the throat has no obstruction, air does not pass through the airway because of the lack of signals from the central nervous system of the brain in the respiratory center. If CSA develops, the blood oxygen levels fall below normal many times during the night, causing heavy snoring and disruptive sleep episodes. With CSA, the blood oxygen levels could fall to dangerously low levels. The regular CPAP machine won't help for this type of sleep apnea.
3. Mixed Sleep Apnea	In mixed sleep apnea, both obstructive sleep apnea (OSA) and central sleep apnea (CSA) episodes occur simultaneously during sleep, making the patient's sickness more traumatic. Only through an overnight sleep study in a sleep clinic, a person can be diagnosed with mixed sleep apnea.
4. Complex Sleep Apnea	In complex sleep apnea, both obstructive sleep apnea (OSA) and central sleep apnea (CSA) episodes occur simultaneously during sleep, making the patient's sickness more traumatic. After a person's OSA is treated with the CPAP machine, the OSA episodes disappear but the CSA episo des starts occurring, making the patient's sickness more complex to understand. A person can be diagnosed with complex sleep apnea only in a well-equipped sleep lab by a sleep specialist.

SYMPTOMS OF SLEEP APNEA [11, 12, 13, 14, 15, 16, 17, 18, 19, 20, 21, 22]

Table 2.2 Symptoms of sleep apnea.

Sleep apnea develops due to airway blockage in the throat, and causes low blood-oxygen levels while sleeping (SpO2 level falls below normal), and affects the heart and brain function either moderately or severely, leading to cognitive deficits.
As a result, a person with sleep apnea feels some or all of the following symptoms:

- Loud snoring, sudden gasping or a choking sound during sleep
- Observed episodes of stopped breathing during the sleep
- Abrupt awakenings accompanied by gasping or choking
- Night sweats and frequent urination in the night (Nocturia)
- Waking up suddenly, sometimes with a racing heart and shortness of breath
- Waking up with dry mouth
- Waking up tired because of insufficient sleep
- Tiredness and exhaustion during the day
- Drowsiness and fatigue during the day
- Poor concentration, and impairment of intellectual capacity
- Falling asleep unexpectedly during the day
- Early morning headache
- Disoriented, act grumpy, impatient, forgetful and moody in the day
- Difficulty concentrating during the day, poor performance at work
- Sudden mood changes, depression or irritability
- Decreased libido, erectile dysfunction, and/or impotence
- High blood pressure, depression, memory loss, and irritability
- Weight gain, obesity or heaviness
- Falling asleep while working, watching television or even while driving a vehicle
  Did you know sleep apnea sufferers caused (and are still causing) car crashes?

CAUSES OF SLEEP APNEA [11, 12, 13, 14, 15, 16, 17, 18, 19, 20, 21, 22]

- **Obesity is the major cause of obstructive sleep apnea (OSA)**. Obesity causes sleep apnea. At the same time, untreated sleep apnea worsens obesity. Which obviously means that the sleep apnea and obesity go hand in hand and influence one another, and worsen the sleep disorder by simultaneously gaining more weight. Obstructive sleep apnea has close association with obesity. When someone is obese, fat cells infiltrate neck and throat tissues so that they lose tone and are more likely to collapse. The neck and chin become enlarged and press on the throat when the person is lying down. Excess fat compresses the chest and makes it difficult to inhale deeply. Finally, too much visceral fat (internal abdominal fat) pushes up on the diaphragm, the sheet of muscular tissue between the abdomen and the chest. As a result, this sleep disorder prevents deep inhalation, lowering the blood oxygen levels (SpO2) significantly. [11, 12]

- **When a person is overweight or obese, the muscles in the back of the throat relax too much, and block the airway**. When the muscles relax, the airway narrows, obstructing the breathing for 10 seconds or longer. This in turn lowers the oxygen percentage saturation in your blood (SpO2 level) to below normal, and causes a buildup of carbon dioxide, thereby causing the obstructive sleep apnea (OSA). Your brain senses this impaired breathing and briefly rouses you from sleep so that you can reopen your airway.

The Oxygen Desaturation Index (ODI) is the number of times per hour the SpO2 level drops by at least 4% (used to be 3%) and stays there for at least 10 seconds. ODI is briefly described as "Desaturation Events or Episodes per Hour." This activity of sleep apnea events or episodes repeats and continues throughout the night. When this activity repeats itself 5 times or more per hour, you develop mild sleep apnea. When this activity repeats itself 15 times or more per hour, you develop moderate sleep apnea. And when this activity repeats itself 30 times or more per hour, you develop severe sleep apnea. [16]

⦾ **Anatomical Factors Cause Sleep Apnea:** The following anatomical abnormalities (which can be seen in a head radiograph) cause obstructive sleep apnea: [14, 15]
♦ Small jaw,
♦ An narrow airway opening in the throat,
♦ Large or long tongue,
♦ Deviated septum,
♦ Swollen tonsils or adenoids,
♦ Enlarged uvula (the small tissue that dangles in the center of your throat),
♦ Too much tissue in the throat, unusual blockages in the mouth, nose and throat.

⦾ **Neck Circumference** [11, 12]
♦ neck circumference of 17 inches or more for men,
♦ neck circumference of 16 inches or more for women,

⦾ **Smoking:** Research showed that smokers are three times more prone to suffering from sleep apnea as compared to non-smokers. Smoking increases inflammation and fluid retention in the upper airway, thereby blocking the inhaled air flow into the lungs. As a result, the SpO2 level goes down during sleep. [14, 15]

⦾ **Alcohol Consumption:** Avoid alcohol, tranquilizers, sedatives, and sleeping pills. Alcohol consumption relaxes the soft tissue of the muscles in the back of your throat, which makes it collapse easily, thereby blocking the airway when you fall asleep. As a result, the SpO2 level goes down during sleep. [14, 15]

⦾ **Heredity or Family History Plays An Important Role.** The defects associated with the function of the throat muscles and blockages are duplicated from parents to children. If one of your parents or siblings suffered from sleep apnea, you are also more likely to have sleep apnea. [14, 15]

⦾ **Sleeping on Your Back** can also cause your airway to become blocked or narrowed, developing obstructive sleep apnea. Side sleeping keeps your airway open. [21]

⦾ **Central Sleep Apnea is another sleep disorder during which breathing can stop**. It occurs when the brain temporarily stops sending signals to the muscles that control breathing. [20]

⦾ **Nasal Congestion.** People (mostly children) whose ability to breathe through the nose is reduced because of congestion are more likely to experience obstructive sleep apnea. [21]

⦾ **Hormone Abnormalities.** Hormone conditions like hypothyroidism (underactive thyroid) and acromegaly (excess growth hormone) may increase the risk of obstructive sleep apnea by causing swelling of tissue near the airway and/or contributing to a person's risk of obesity. [21]

30

RISK FACTORS, LONG-TERM SIDE EFFECTS AND COMPLICATIONS
[11, 12, 13, 14, 15, 16, 17, 18, 19, 20, 21, 22, 23, 24]

Table 2.3 Risk factors, long-term side effects, and complications of sleep apnea.

Sleep Apnea is Dangerous! It Could Develop The Following Health Risks and Complications! Take Action Now!	
1. Low Blood Oxygen Level (Low SpO2)	17. Pressure Changes in the Heart
2. Repeated Episodes of Low SpO2 (Hypoxia)	18. Heart Attack
3. Excess Body Weight Gain & Obesity	19. Congestive Heart Failure
4. Difficulty to Lose Weight	20. Arrhythmia or Atrial Fibrillation (an irregular heartbeat)
5. Type 2 Diabetes	21. Cardiomyopathy (enlargement of the muscle tissue of the heart)
6. High Blood Pressure (Hypertension)	22. Brain Fog & Brain Infection
7. Difficulty to Treat High Blood Pressure	23. Multiple Sclerosis
8. Headaches	24. Presence of a Tumor
9. Drowsiness While Walking & Driving	25. Stroke
10. Daytime Fatigue & Sleepiness	26. Memory Loss and Dementia
11. Chronic Insomnia at Night	27. Lung Hypertension
12. Chronic Nasal Congestion at Night	28. Eye Problems
13. Unable to Focus and Thrive	29. Sleep Apnea is Linked to Cancer
14. Anxiety & Depression	30. Many Other Strange Problems
15. Erectile Dysfunction & Impotence	
16. Alteration in Craniofacial Structures	

COMPLICATIONS OF OBESITY [25]

Table 2.4 Complications of obesity.

Sleep Apnea and Obesity Influence One Another, and Develp The Following Complications! Take Action Now!
1. Obesity Causes Sleep Apnea
2. Sleep Apnea Causes Obesity
3. Type 2 Diabetes
4. Pancreatitis
5. Heart Disease
6. Arthritis
7. Gout
8. Gallstones
9. Lung Disease
10. Liver Disease
11. Cancer
12. Stroke

SLEEP APNEA VERSUS COPD [26, 27, 28, 29, 30]

While this book's purpose is to teach all about sleep apnea, this section talks about COPD.

WHAT IS COPD?
• COPD stands for chronic obstructive pulmonary disease. COPD is closely related to cigarette exposure in those who smoke or those who have secondhand exposure to smoke. Long-term exposure to air pollution (including smoke, dust, fumes and chemicals) also causes COPD, and directly damages the lungs.

• COPD causes permanent damage to the lungs and worsen breathing day by day, and develops airway obstruction. A person with advanced COPD may be unable to climb the stairs, and may not even cook. They may need medications and supplementary oxygen.

COPD STATISTICS
• More than 65 million people around the world have moderate or severe COPD, and experts predict that this number will continue to rise worldwide over the next 50 years.

• In 2015, 3.2 million people died from COPD worldwide, an increase of 11.6% compared with 1990. During that same time period, the prevalence of COPD increased by 44.2% to 174.5 million individuals.

• In the United States alone, at least 16 million adults have COPD. The American Lung Association (ALA) thinks there may be as many as 24 million American adults living with COPD.

MORE ABOUT COPD
• Obstructive sleep apnea (OSA) occurs when the breathing stops and starts repeatedly throughout the night, thereby creating the episodes of apneas and hypopnes. Chronic obstructive pulmonary disease (COPD) is a group of lung conditions that make breathing difficult by blocking airflow in the lungs as the lungs structure many have been seriously damaged. These two conditions are different, but they may occur together and worsen each other's symptoms. When OSA and COPD occur simultaneously, overlap syndrome (OS) develops. Many people suffer from overlap syndrome (OS).

• The SpO2 level drops to below normal even during the day if you have COPD. That is why, COPD patients keep a spot check oximeter at home and monitor their SpO2 level during the day whenever they feel low in oxygen level. But if you have sleep apnea, the SpO2 level drops to below normal mostly during the night when you fall asleep. In that case you cannot use spot check oximeter, you need to use an oximeter for continuous monitoring, and do the "overnight pulse oximetry test," upload the data to your computer, and find out your oxygen desaturation index (events per hour) to find out the severity of the sleep apnea (mild, moderate or severe).

• There is no cure for COPD, but the symptoms can be minimized and managed by appropriate treatments. However the obstructive sleep apnea can be cured and even reversed by losing excess body weight (if there are no serious blockages and obstructions in the throat, mouth and nose).

• The symptoms of both OSA and COPD can be minimized and managed with the help of CPAP therapy or BiPAP therapy as is the most common treatment being used.

TYPES OF COPD

COPD is associated with two types (i) Emphysema and (ii) Chronic Bronchitis.
Emphysema damages the air sacs in the lungs and makes them less efficient.
Chronic bronchitis causes inflammation of the airways called bronchial tubes, which can result in a buildup of mucus.

SYMPTOMS OF COPD

- Chronic coughing with or without sputum
- Wheezing: Wheezing is a high-pitched whistling sound made while breathing
  It's often associated with difficulty breathing and painful breathing
- Constant tiredness, fatigue, and lack of energy
- Shortness of breath (an inability to breath easily or take a deep breath)
- Frequent respiratory infections
- Rapid heart beat
- Reduced mental alertness

DIAGNOSIS

- By asking questions and from the signs and symptoms a patient is being experienced, the doctor identifies the disease, and orders further tests.
- Spirometry test measures the amount and speed of airflow during a short breath. The person blows hard into a tube attached to a device called spirometer, which gives the reading. The test results show the abnormal air flow rate through the lungs.
- Your doctor may also order a fast and painless imaging test such as a chest x-ray or a chest CT (a high resolution computed tomography) to see damages in your lungs.

TREATMENT OF COPD

- Stop smoking immediately
- Use CPAP therapy or BiPAP therapy every single night
  (Never sleep without hooking up to your CPAP or BiPAP machine)
- Use supplemental oxygen and medications if necessary
- Work out every day in the gym
- Learn and practice how to boost exercise tolerance
- Join a pulmonary rehabilitation course
- Do breathing exercises daily to improve lungs function
- Practice yoga and meditation focussing on breathing

SURGERY

- LUNGS TRANSPLANTATION (a single or double lung transplant)
- A bullectomy to remove the larger air sacs that affect breathing
- The removal of damaged lung tissue, known as lung volume reduction surgery
- The placement of endobronchial valves in the part of the lung with the most damage
  (A specially trained surgeon places endobronchial valves)

BLOOD OXYGEN SATURATION (SpO2) [31, 32, 33]

VERY IMPORTANT: If you are diagnosed with sleep apnea, you should understand thoroughly what oxygen saturation in the blood (SpO2) is, and what oxygen desaturation in the blood is. If you have sleep apnea, your blood oxygen level falls below normal throughout the night when you sleep because of the airway blockage and simultaneous snoring and, as a result, you will face severe health complications. So be prepared to battle this challenge. But first, you must learn and understand what exactly the SpO2 level is with a clear concept.

Blood carries oxygen from the lungs to the trillions of body cells where it is burned. But the oxygen could react quickly in the blood and burn prematurely before it reaches the trillions of body's cells. This premature burning is prevented by a protein molecule called "hemoglobin" present in the red blood cells.[31] The blood in the human body contains about 30 trillion red blood cells. Each red blood cell has about 270 million protein molecules. Each protein molecule represents a ring composed of carbon, nitrogen and hydrogen atoms. This ring floats in the bloodstream and a cluster of 4 iron atoms that sit in the center of each ring protect a pair of oxygen atoms from premature burning. This incredibly-designed protein molecule is called "hemoglobin." [31]

Oxygen molecules are carried throughout the body through blood, attached to hemoglobin molecules. [16] One hemoglobin molecule can carry a maximum of 4 oxygen molecules. If all 4 molecules of oxygen are perfectly attached to one hemoglobin molecule, the oxygen is said to be one 100% saturated. Oxygen saturation is usually refereed to as SpO2 and is expressed in percentage (%).[32, 33]

• If 3 oxygen molecules are attached to one hemoglobin molecule, then the oxygen is said to be 75% (3/4 = 0.75 = 75%) saturated.
• If 2 oxygen molecules are attached to one hemoglobin molecule, then the oxygen is said to be 50% (2/4 = 0.50 = 50%) saturated.
• If 3.8 oxygen molecules are precisely attached to one hemoglobin molecule, then the oxygen is said to be 95% (3.8/4 = 0.95 = 95%) saturated, and so on.
Normal Oxygen Saturation Level (SpO2) at sea level is between 96% and 99%.

Table 2.5 How to understand blood oxygen saturation (SpO2).

Oxygen Saturation	Number of Oxygen molecules Attached to Hemoglobin
4/4 = 100%	All 4 oxygen molecules are attached to one hemoglobin molecule.
3/4 = 75%	3 oxygen molecules are attached to one hemoglobin molecule.
2/4 = 50%	2 oxygen molecules are attached to one hemoglobin molecule.
1/4 = 25%	1 oxygen molecules are attached to one hemoglobin molecule.
3.96/4 = 99%	3.96 oxygen molecules are attached to one hemoglobin molecule.
3.92/4 = 98%	3.92 oxygen molecules are attached to one hemoglobin molecule.
3.88/4 = 97%	3.88 oxygen molecules are attached to one hemoglobin molecule.
3.84/4 = 96%	3.84 oxygen molecules are attached to one hemoglobin molecule.
3.80/4 = 95%	3.80 oxygen molecules are attached to one hemoglobin molecule.
3.76/4 = 94%	3.76 oxygen molecules are attached to one hemoglobin molecule.
3.72/4 = 93%	3.72 oxygen molecules are attached to one hemoglobin molecule.
3.68/4 = 92%	3.68 oxygen molecules are attached to one hemoglobin molecule.
3.64/4 = 91%	3.64 oxygen molecules are attached to one hemoglobin molecule.
3.60/4 = 90%	3.60 oxygen molecules are attached to one hemoglobin molecule.
	and so on....

SPOT CHECK OXIMETERS

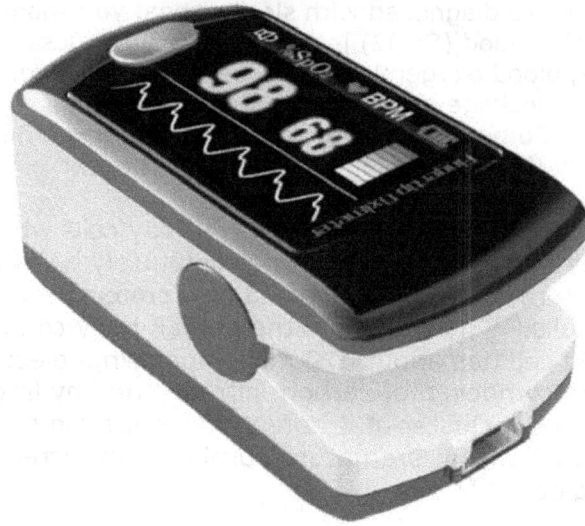

SPOT CHECK FINGER-PULSE OXIMETER [34]
SpO2 = 98%; Pulse Rate = 68

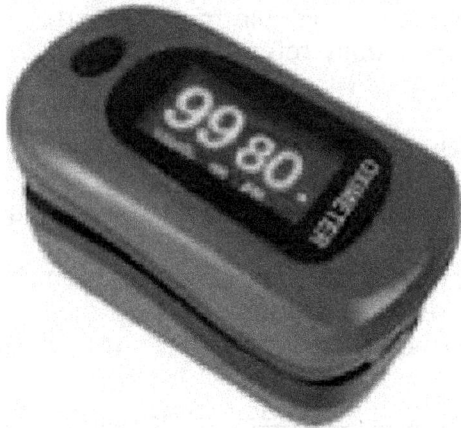

SPOT CHECK FINGER-PULSE OXIMETER
SpO2 = 99%; Pulse Rate = 80

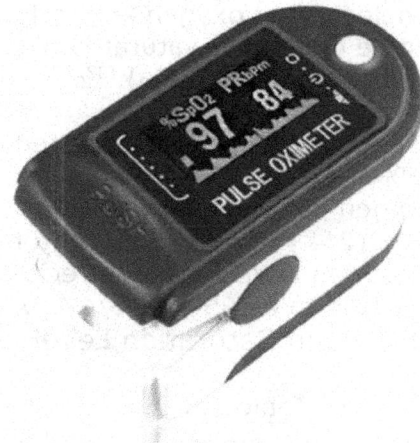

SPOT CHECK FINGER-PULSE OXIMETER
SpO2 = 97%; Pulse Rate = 84

Spot Check Finger-Pulse Oximeters are used to monitor the SpO2 level (percentage saturation of oxygen in the blood) instantly to evaluate a patient's condition. If there is a lack of oxygen in the blood, your body tissues will not be oxygenated properly and can be hazardous to your health. By simply inserting the finger into the sensor probe of the oximeter, a person's SpO2 level can be monitored instantly, and find out if there is abnormal SpO2 level. Many athletes and pilots who travel at high altitudes use this unit to instantly monitor and know their SpO2 level. This spot check oximeter is also used in the hospital emergency rooms to evaluate the patient's respiratory or cardiac problems and sleep disorder concerns. Many patients, especially those who suffer from COPD and other sleep disorders, also use the finger-pulse oximeter at home to monitor SpO2 level on a daily basis. However this kind of spot check oximeter cannot be used to store data so that you can look back and examine the data to understand the severity of your sleep disorder. More importantly, it cannot be used to find out the Desaturation Index (the number of events per hour during the night) of a sleep apnea patient.

Courtesy of 123CHECKUP.Com
Figure 2.6 Spot check finger-pulse oximeter.

THE PRINCIPLE OF FINGER-PULSE OXIMETER

A pulse oximeter is a non-invasive photoelectric device specially designed to monitor SpO2 level. A reusable probe can be placed on the finger or a single use tape probe is placed on the earlobe or finger. It works by passing a beam of red and infrared light through a pulsating capillary bed. The ratio of red to infrared blood light transmitted gives a measure of the oxygen saturation of the blood (SpO2). The oximeter works on the principle that the oxygenated blood is a brighter color of red than the deoxygenated blood, which is more blue-purple. First, the oximeter measures the sum of the intensity of both shades of red, representing the fractions of the blood with and without oxygen. The oximeter detects the pulse, and then subtracts the intensity of color detected when the pulse is absent. The remaining intensity of color represents only the oxygenated red blood. This is displayed on the electronic screen as a percentage of oxygen saturation in the blood (SpO2). [35, 36]

OXYGEN DESATURATION INDEX (ODI) | DESATURATION INDEX

Oxygen Desaturation Event or Episode: Drop in SpO2 level by at least 4% (recently it was reduced to 3%) for a minimum duration of 10 seconds. For example the SpO2 level dropped from 99% to 96% during sleep, and stayed at 96% for 10 seconds or more, it is counted as one "oxygen desaturation event or episode (or one apnea)." Those drops may continue during the night, and are called "oxygen desaturations," and those drops can be monitored by a pulse oximeter . [37]

Oxygen Desaturation Index (ODI), or simply called Desaturation Index, is the number of times the SpO2 level drops per hour by at least 4% (recently it was reduced to 3%) and stays like that for at least 10 seconds. [35] The ODI is also measured in the sleep study laboratories by carefully generating diagnostic polysomnogram, in which a sleep apnea patient is hooked up with many sensors and then the patient is asked to sleep overnight.

Normal/Healthy SpO2 level at sea level should be between 96% and 99%.
The severity of the sleep apnea is determined from the reduction in the SpO2 levels, and the reductions are classified as follows: [37]

Table 2.6 Assessment guidelines of sleep apnea using desaturation index.

SpO2 Level	Desaturation Index	Assessment
(%)	(Events/hr)	
96% - 99%	0 - 4	Normal
90% - 95%	5 - 14	Mild Sleep Apnea
80% - 90%	15 - 29	Moderate Sleep Apnea
< 80%	≥ 30	Severe Sleep Apnea

APNEA HYPOPNEA INDEX (AHI)

The Apnea Hypopnea Index (AHI) is also used to indicate the severity of obstructive sleep apnea. Apnea occurs when the stoppage of breathing developed due to complete obstruction of airflow from nose to lungs. Hypopnea occurs when shallow or slow breathing is developed due to partial obstruction in the airway of the throat. Hypopnea is less severe compared to apnea. Both conditions have similar causes and symptoms, and both conditions are to be treated in the same way. The severity of the sleep apnea is determined from the reductions in the SpO2 levels, and the reductions are classified as follows:[38]

Table 2.7 Assessment guidelines of sleep apnea using AHI.

SpO2 Level	AHI	Assessment
(%)	(Events/hr)	
96% - 99%	0 - 4	Normal
90% - 95%	5 - 14	Mild Sleep Apnea
80% - 90%	15 - 29	Moderate Sleep Apnea
< 80%	≥ 30	Severe Sleep Apnea

FINGER PULSE OXIMETERS FOR CONTINUOUS MONITORING [39, 40]
TO DO THE OVERNIGHT PULSE OXIMETRY TEST FOR SLEEP APNEA

If you have sleep apnea, the soft tissue of your throat muscle relaxes and blocks your airway whenever you fall asleep, and as a result your SpO2 level drops. When you are awake, your airway is not blocked so your SpO2 level stays normal. So if you use spot check oximeter when you are awake, your SpO2 level is always normal (unless you have COPD). Therefore your SpO2 level must be monitored continuously using a device such as Philips Respironics Oximeter, Nonin Oximeter, or ResMed Apnealink Air Device so that you can look back the stored data and find out how your SpO2 level has been dropping and fluctuating throughout the night whenever you sleep.

As mentioned earlier, a spot check pulse oximeter gives the SpO2 level at that instant only whenever you monitor, but it does not tell you the whole story about your disease or sleep disorder. A spot check oximeter cannot be used to store data so that you can look back and examine the data to understand the severity of your sleep disorder.

Therefore it is important that you should purchase a device for continuous monitoring and learn how to use it confidently at the comfort of your home. You must learn how to find out the Desaturation Index (events/hr), minimum SpO2, mean SpO2, maximum SpO2 and SpO2 versus time chart by doing the overnight pulse oximetry test. A high-precision Philips Respironics Oximeter or Nonin Oximeter (shown below) would serve this purpose.

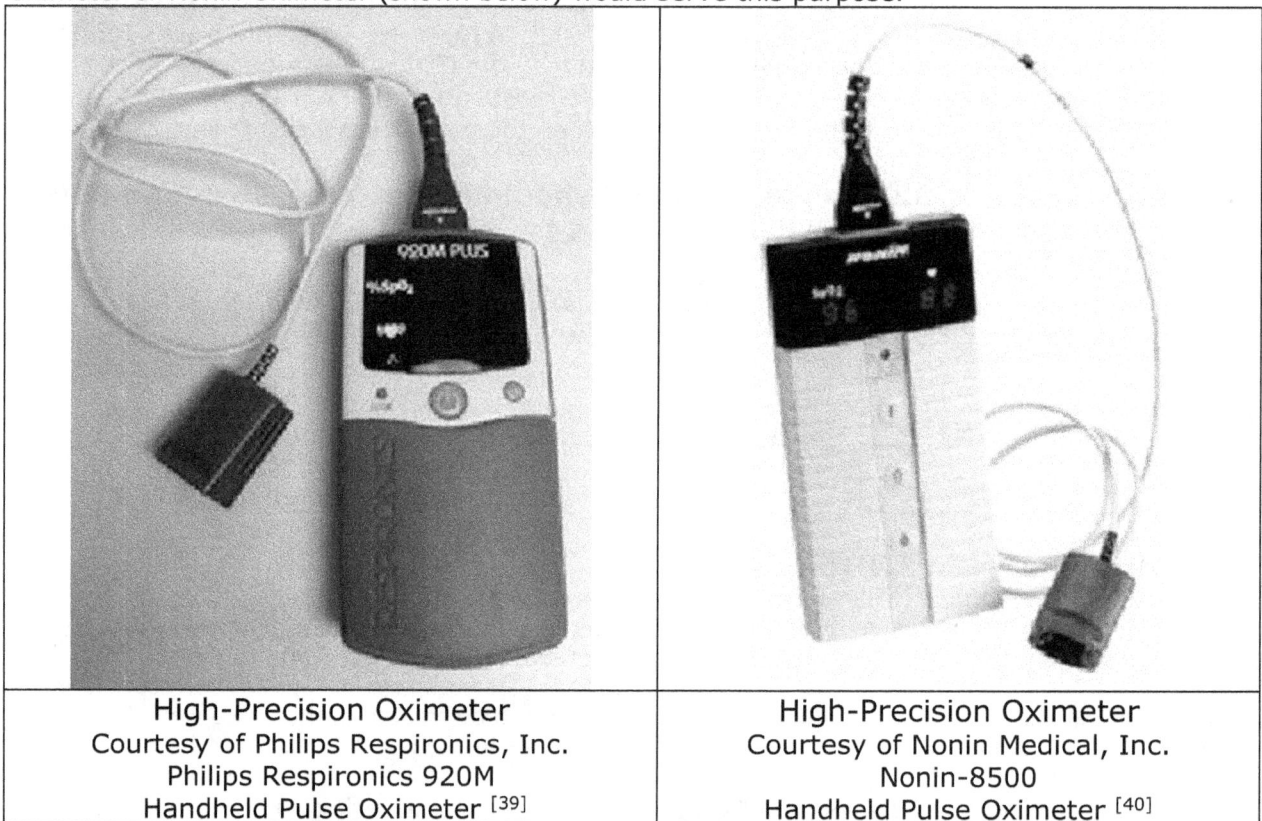

High-Precision Oximeter	High-Precision Oximeter
Courtesy of Philips Respironics, Inc.	Courtesy of Nonin Medical, Inc.
Philips Respironics 920M	Nonin-8500
Handheld Pulse Oximeter [39]	Handheld Pulse Oximeter [40]

Figure 2.7 High-Precision Pulse oximeter for continuous monitoring to do overnight pulse oximetry test.

1. You can borrow this kind of pulse oximeter (Respironics or Nonin Oximeter) from your doctor's sleep clinic or from the CPAP vendor where you purchased your CPAP machine. Or you can purchase it online, own it, and do your own test. It could cost from $2000 to $5000.

2. Make sure the batteries are new and would last for 2 to 3 nights continuously before you use it. Make sure the oximeter is in good working condition as those doctor's clinics and those CPAP vendors lend the same oximeter over and over again to many patients. So it is your duty to make sure that the oximeter is reliable and is in a good working condition before start using it for the "overnight pulse oximetry test." It would be a good idea to do the overnight oximetry test with two different companies and make sure the results match.

3. When you are ready to start the test at 9 pm or 10 pm, plug in the sensor to the oximeter and insert your finger into the probe. Tighten the probe very gently with a rubberband, or tighten the sensor cable with a tape so that your finger would not slip out during the sleep. And then turn on the oximeter by pressing the on-button.

4. Then the oximeter starts monitoring, recording and displaying the SpO2 level and pulse rate. After some 30 to 60 seconds, the display disappears automatically, but it would still be monitoring, recording and storing your SpO2 values and pulse rate values in its memory continuously throughout the night. You can continue using this oximeter throughout the night until the next morning (at around 7 am or whenever you wake up). If your oxygen level (SpO2 leve) fall below normal or too low, you can see those dangerous levels early in the next morning by uploading the data to your computer. You must sleep at least 4 hours, or the software would generate wrong results.

5. When you go to the bathroom during the night, you just place the oximeter into your shirt's pocket of your pajama so that you would not drop it in the bathroom (do not remove the finger from the probe).

6. After completing the test, press the off-button and it will stop recording. Next morning, return this pulse oximeter to your provider (your sleep clinic doctor or the CPAP vendor) where they would upload the data to a computer, and the software would calculate and display the following results of the sleep apnea patient who took the test:

- Desaturation Index (number of desaturation events/hr),
- Minimum SpO2, Mean SpO2 and Maximum SpO2,
- SpO2 Vs Time Chart, and Pulse Rate Vs Time Chart.

7. From the aforementioned information, it is possible to know the severity of the obstructive sleep apnea (mild, moderate or severe) of any person living with sleep apnea symptoms.

8. Get a copy of the test results from your doctor or provider, and try to understand the results, and keep a record of it so that you can always refer to these test results in the future.

9. It is recommended that you should take this "overnight pulse oximetry test" at least once every 6 months, and maintain a progress report of your sleep apnea condition. If you want seriously reverse your obstructive sleep apnea, it is highly recommended that you better purchase this kind of finger pulse oximeter online, own it, and do your own test as frequently as you want.

IMPORTANT NOTE: When taking the "overnight pulse oximetry test," you should not use CPAP therapy (or any other therapy) simultaneously. As a matter of fact, in order to get accurate results, you must discontinue the use of CPAP therapy for at least a week prior to the "overnight pulse oximetry test." Otherwise the use of CPAP therapy influences the true value of your Desturation Index (number of desaturation events per hour), and could generate erroneous or misleading results.

MOST RECENTLY: The aforementioned two pulse oximeters (Philips Respironics Oximeter and Nonin Oximeter) are now replaced by a more comprehensive device called "ResMed ApneaLink™ Air Home Sleep Testing Device," which can be borrowed from a local CPAP vendor or from any local sleep clinic. "ResMed ApneaLink™ Air Home Sleep Testing Device" is explained below.

ResMed ApneaLink™ Air Home Sleep Testing Device
MOST RECENT CONTINUOUS MONITORING DEVICE TO DO THE OVERNIGHT PULSE OXIMETRY DIAGNOSTIC TEST FOR SLEEP APNEA

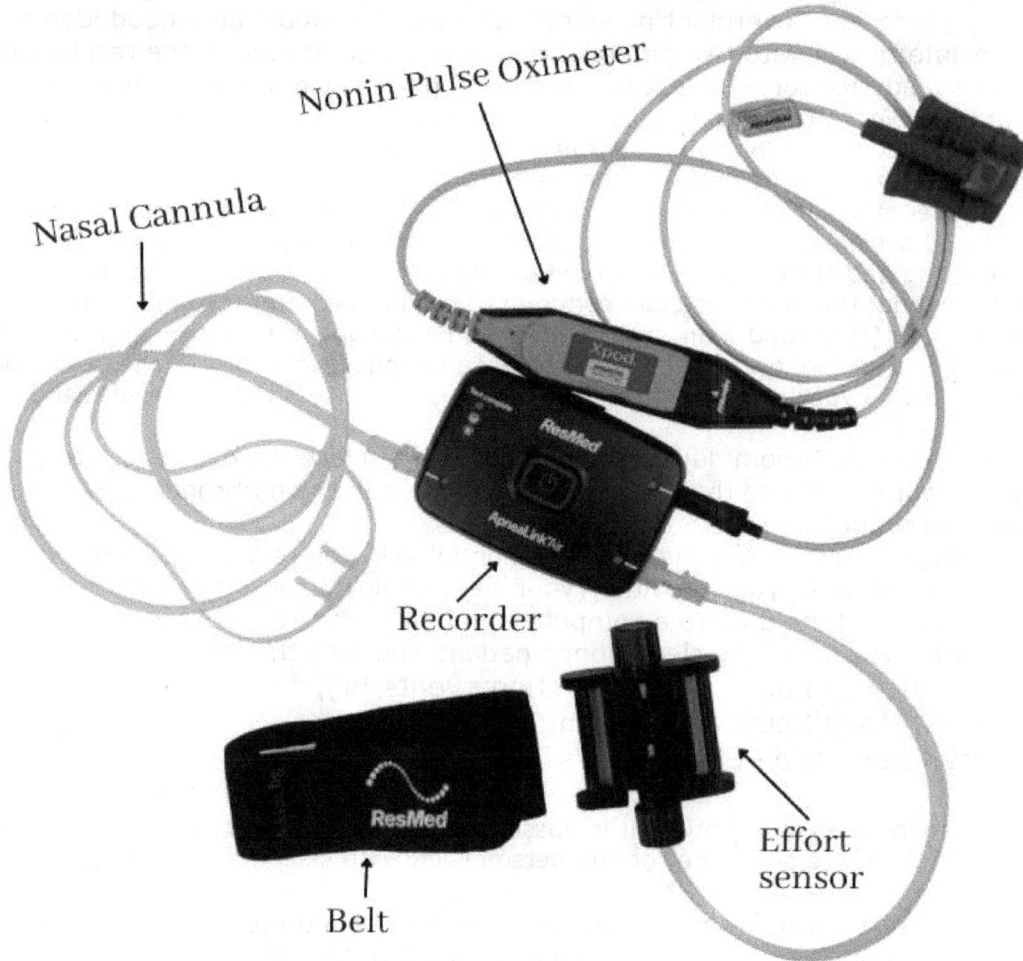

Courtesy of ResMed
Figure 2.8 ResMed ApneaLink™ Air Home Sleep Testing High-Precision Device.

ResMed ApneaLink™ Air Home Sleep Testing Device [41, 42, 43]

It is used to do comprehensive overnight and non-invasive diagnostic test (Level III test) in order to determine if you suffer from sleep apnea or sleep disorder breathing. It measures 5 different variables for further clinical investigation, or when a basic oximetry screening test is deemed to be inconclusive. This device is offered for free to all sleep apnea patients. Being a cost effective home sleep testing device, the ResMed ApneaLink™ Air Home Sleep Testing Device is capable of recording up to five channels of information: respiratory effort, pulse, oxygen saturation, nasal flow and snoring. The Device comes with the following components to be assembled together:

(i) ApneaLink Air Recorder (the black box with ResMed Logo on it),
(ii) Black-Colored Belt,
(iii) Effort Sensor (It monitors chest expansion and contraction),
(iv) Nasal Cannula (It is a transparent long narrow hose, and it monitors the airflow of breathing, snoring volume & respiratory effort during sleep), and
(v) Nonin Pulse Oximeter or SAT Probe (It is a small rectangular blue bar, and it monitors Desaturation Index in events per/hr, minimum SpO2, mean SpO2 and maximum SpO2).

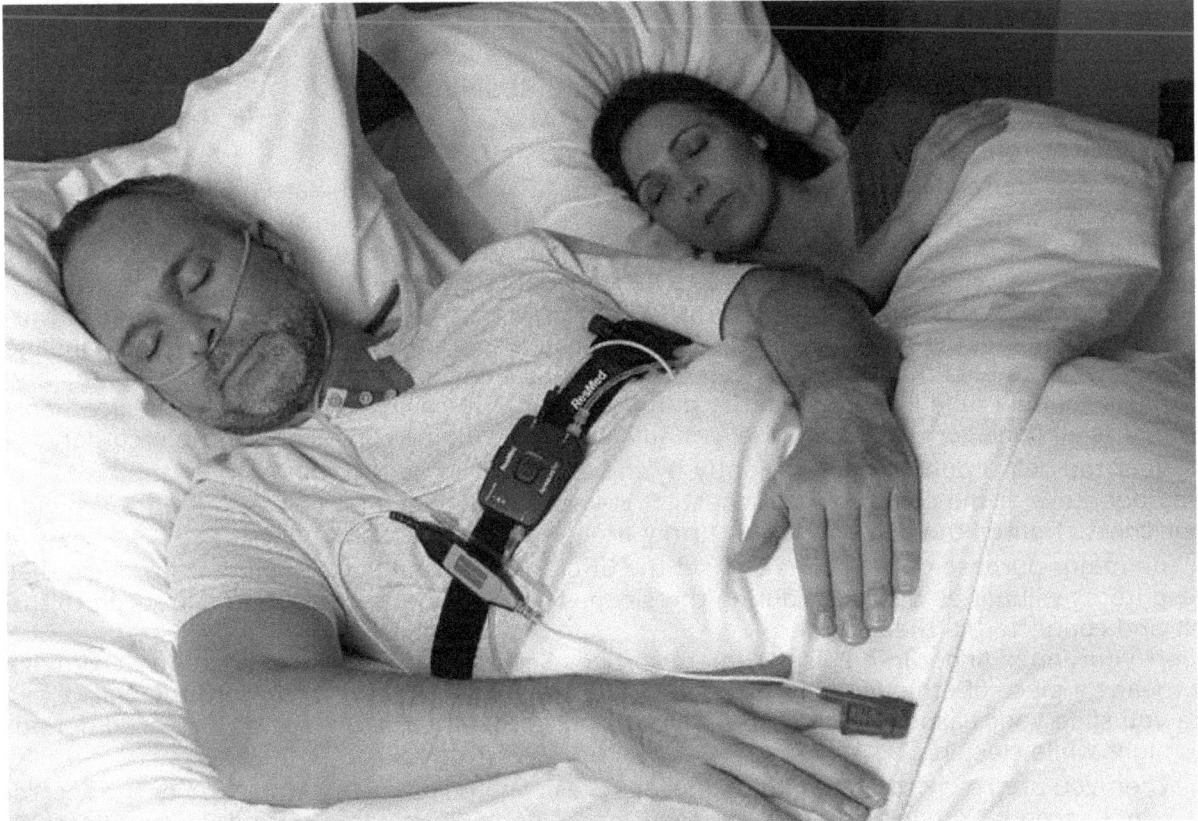

Courtesy of ResMed

Figure 2.9 A sleep apnea patient is taking the overnight pulse oximetry test at home using "ResMed ApneaLink™ Air" device.

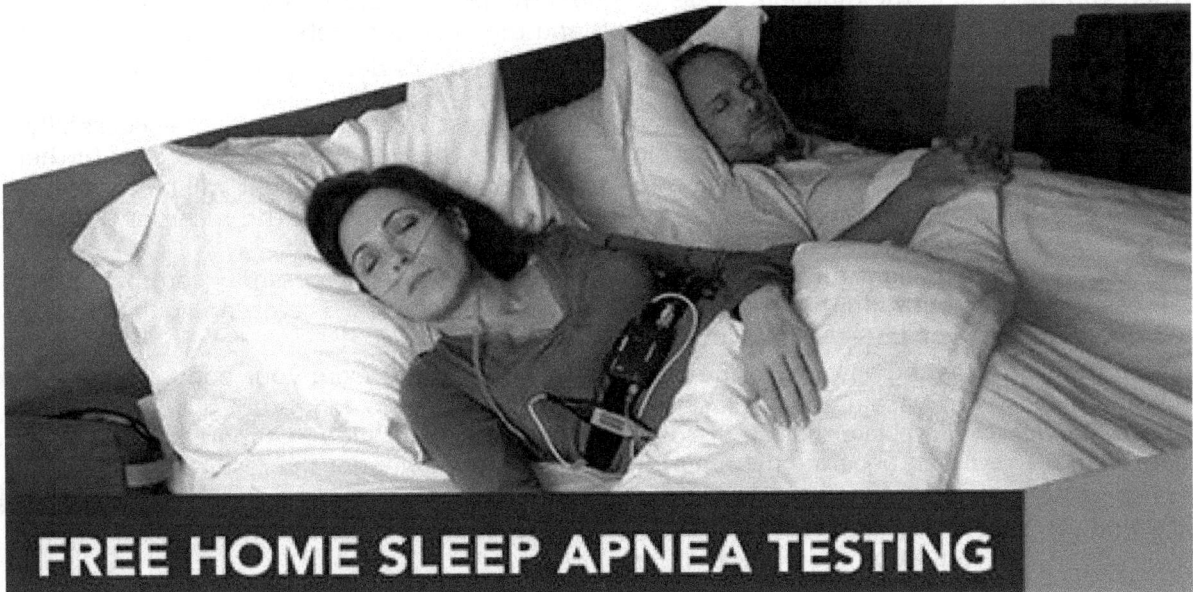

FREE HOME SLEEP APNEA TESTING

Courtesy of ResMed

Figure 2.10 A sleep apnea patient is taking the overnight pulse oximetry test at home using "ResMed ApneaLink™ Air" device.

HOW TO ASSEMBLE AND USE THE RESMED APPNEALINK AIR DEVICE?
HOW TO DO THE OVERNIGHT PULSE OXIMETRY DIAGNOSTIC TEST?

Please watch the YouTube video uploaded by ResMed. [44, 45]
https://www.youtube.com/watch?v=awa4z2fFn7A
https://www.youtube.com/watch?v=UEdGJp5fL40

a. When you are ready to take the overnight sleep test at your home late evening around 9 pm or 10 pm, wear the nasal cannula by following instructions provided in the brochure, and by standing in front of a mirror. You need to loop and hang the nasal cannula to your ears and then tighten the loop. Dip the two prongs of the nasal cannula into your nostrils facing downwards, and tighten the loop again by pulling the slider up towards your chin. If the two prongs of the nasal cannula do not stay in the nostrils of your nose, use a medical tape or adhesive bandages on the cheeks to hold them in your nostrils. When nasal canula is properly worn insert the end of the nasal cannula tube into the recorder and tighten it by turning it in the clockwise direction. When it is all done correctly, the nasal cannula sensor would be connected to the recorder.

b. Wear the belt around the chest tightly by means of Velcro so that the AppneaLink Air Recorder stays at the center of your chest. It is very simple belt with velcro that goes around your chest. Tighten the belt and lock it firmly around your chest using Velcro.

c. The major purpose of the belt is to hold the Effort Sensor and Pulse Oximeter firmly so that these items will not be displaced during the sleep. The Effort Sensor is already attached to the belt and connected to the recorder.
Insert your index finger into Pulse Oximeter probe. Secure the long wire of the Pulse Oximeter by means a piece of athletic tape if needed. Slide the pulse oximeter firmly into the belt (exactly like you slide your ballpoint pen into your shirt's pocket) so that it will not be displaced during the night while sleeping.

d. When you are ready to go to bed and sleep, press and hold the Power-Button of the recorder for 2 to 3 seconds. You will immediately see 3 green lights illuminated. These 3 green lights represent the 3 sensors (pulse oximeter sensor, effort sensor and nasal cannula sensor). If any light is RED, check the corresponding line of connection, and make sure the sensor is connected to the recorder correctly.

e. When you wake up in the morning, press and hold the power-button of the recorder for 2 to 3 seconds. Then the 3 green lights will be turned off and the Test Complete Light turns green if the test was completed successfully. It is important that you must sleep at least 4 hours to successfully complete the test.
(i) If the Test Complete Light turns RED, that means your test was not completed successfully. You need to repeat the test in the following night or contact the Healthcare Provider for further assistance. Press and hold the Power-Button for 2 to 3 seconds, the RED light will be turned off. When you get RED light, you should replace two triple-A batteries so that the recorder will work well when you do the test in the following night.
(ii) If the Test Complete Light turned GREEN, that means you have successfully completed the test. Press the power-button of the recorder again for 2 to 3 seconds. The green light will be turned off. And then whole recorder will be turned off.

f. Detach the whole testing assembly (the belt and Nasal Cannula) from your body. You can detach and dispose the Nasal Canula. Place all the items in the bag, and return the bag to your Healthcare Provider who will later upload the data to a computer, the software program would analyse the data from the recorder, generate the report into PSD file, and print out the results if needed.

g. You should eagerly ask and request your Healthcare Provider to email you a copy of your sleep test results. And you should read the report and understand the following important test results:
- Desaturation Index (events/hr),
- Minimum SpO2, Mean SpO2 and Maximum SpO2,
- SpO2 Vs Time Chart, and Pulse Rate Vs Time Chart.
- Chest compressions and Snoring Information (if possible).

HOW TO PURCHASE A PULSE OXIMETER FROM RESELLERS? HOW TO TEST THE PULSE OXIMETER YOU PURCHASED BY DOING THE "OVERNIGHT PULSE OXIMETRY TEST" AT HOME?

● <u>Take control of your health into your own hands</u>. Do not depend on hospitals, doctors, therapists, or CPAP vendors who can do the "overnight pulse oximetry test" for you. Instead, do your own test, and learn how to do it confidently on your own.

● Research on the Internet and find out a finger pulse oximeter that can be used to do the "overnight Pulse Oximetry text" at home. Remember that Spot Check Oximeters cannot be used to do the "overnight pulse oximetry test." Talk to the vendors, and purchase a pulse oximeter that can be used for continuous monitoring. Make sure it comes with software.

● Make sure that the device comes with 30-day money back guarantee, and one-year manufacturer's warranty, and that the reseller is reliable with a valid address and phone number.

● <u>Do not purchase a Wrist Pulse Oximeter on eBay.com. You can very well be ripped off</u>. There are many resellers selling unreliable Wrist Pulse Oximeters on eBay.com. Be careful with these resellers. They don't offer any technical support. They are just sales people and don't know anything about the device. If the device does not work, they won't help you.

● If there is light on the device, it doesn't mean that the device is working. If you can monitor SpO2 level instantly (it could be a false reading), it doesn't mean that the device is in good working condition. You should do the "overnight pulse oximetry test," and then take a decision whether or not the device is reliable and trustworthy.

● Make sure that the device comes with software that can be easily installed on your computer. And make sure that the vendor is willing to teach you over the phone how to install the software and how to generate report after doing the "overnight pulse oximetry test," and provide you technical support on troubleshooting.

● <u>VERY IMPORTANT: Borrow a high-precision Nonin Oximeter, Respironics Oximeter, or ResMed ApneaLink Air device from a sleep clinic or from any local CPAP vendor to do the overnight pulse oximetry test</u>.
● <u>Do the overnight pulse oximetry test using both devices at the same time (the high-precision device you borrowed from a sleep clinic or CPAP vendor, and the pulse oximeter you just purchased online) so that you can compare the results from both devices</u>.

● After you take the test overnight using both devices, wake up early in the morning, upload the data from the device you purchased to your computer. The software should generate a report with the following results:
        a. Desaturation Index (events/hr)
        b. Minimum SpO2, Mean SpO2 and Maximum SpO2
        c. SpO2 Vs Time Chart, and Pulse Rate Vs Time Chart
Also get the report of the high-precision device which you borrowed from a sleep clinic or CPAP vendor so that you compare the results obtained from both devices.

● If the results obtained by the device you purchased match well with the results obtained by high-precision oximeter, that means the device you purchased is reliable (keep it!). Up to 10% of error is acceptable. If the error is more than 10%, that means the device you purchased is defective. Return the defective device, and get your money back.

WRIST PULSE OXIMETERS
[LOW-PRESCISION CHEAP OXIMETERS]

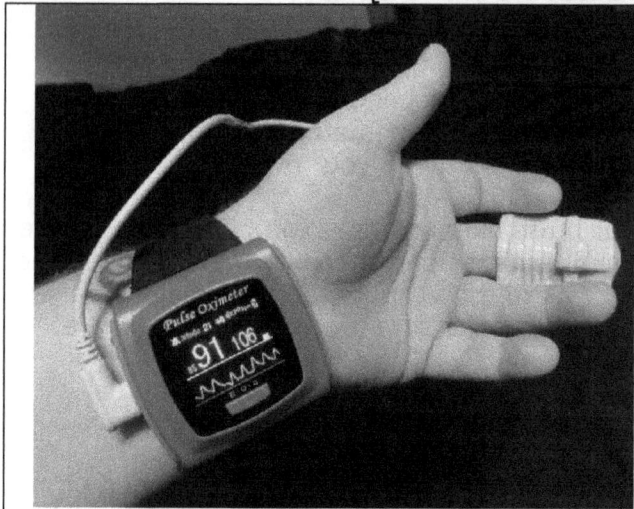

Figure 2.11

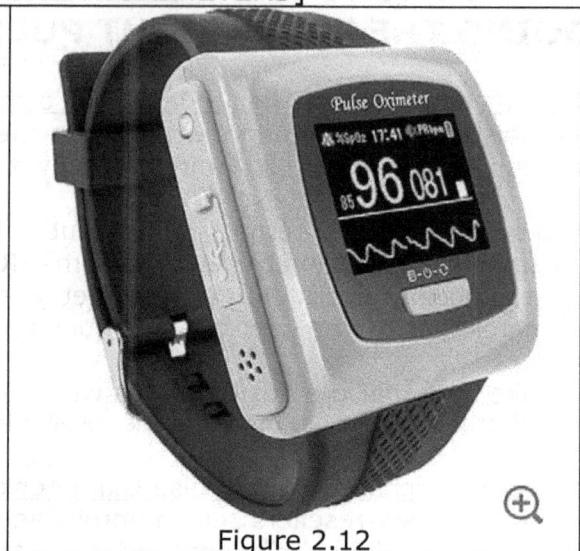

Figure 2.12

Wrist Pulse Oximeter to do the "overnight pulse oximetry test."

THE TRUTH ABOUT WRIST PULSE OXIMETERS:
WRIST PULSE OXIMETERS ARE UNTRUSTWORTHY!

● There are many Wrist Pulse Oximeters being sold online for continuous monitoring. Whether you suffer from sleep apnea or COPD, by wearing this kind of device to your wrist, you can do your own "overnight pulse oximetry test" anytime you want without depending on your sleep clinic doctors, therapists, or CPAP vendors who can do the test for you once a year.

● It would be wonderful if there is such a comfortable mini device available for such a low price ($100 to $200). By self-monitoring frequently, a patient can control and manage in an attempt to improve or even reverse his/her sleep disorder.

● However, before using this kind of low-precision Wrist Pulse Oximeter, please test it by comparing the result (Desaturation Index) with that of a high-precision oximeter. Do the "overnight pulse oximetry test" by sleeping with both devices (high-precision oximeter and low-precision oximeter) on the same night, and compare the result (Desaturation Index) obtained by both devices. If you notice that the low-precision device is giving significant error, please do not use such low-precision device. It could generate misleading results and could put you in the wrong direction.

● **WARNING & CAUTION:** We have tested several Wrist Pulse Oximeters by comparing the test result (Desaturation Index) with that of a high-precision Philips Respironics Pulse Oximeter or Nonin Pulse Oximeter, and we have determined that the Wrist Pulse Oximeter gives an error of 50% to 70%, and therefore it is unreliable and untrustworthy.

LIST OF RESELLERS TO PURCHASE A PULSE OXIMETER

+++

The following resellers sell Nonin Oximeters, Wrist Pulse Oximeters, Spot Check oximeters, and other high-precision oxmeters. Do your own research and purchase an oximeter. Please do not purchase CONTEC Wrist Pulse Oximeter from these resellers, which is not reliable and generates false results (we have already tested one).

+++

TURNER MEDICAL

35 Highwood Cir.

Colchester, CT 06415

Toll Free: 1-866-778-5890

Fax: 860-812-2087

Email: orders@turnermedical.com

https://www.turnermedical.com/default.asp

https://www.turnermedical.com/SPOT_CHECK_PULSE_OXIMETER_s/70.htm

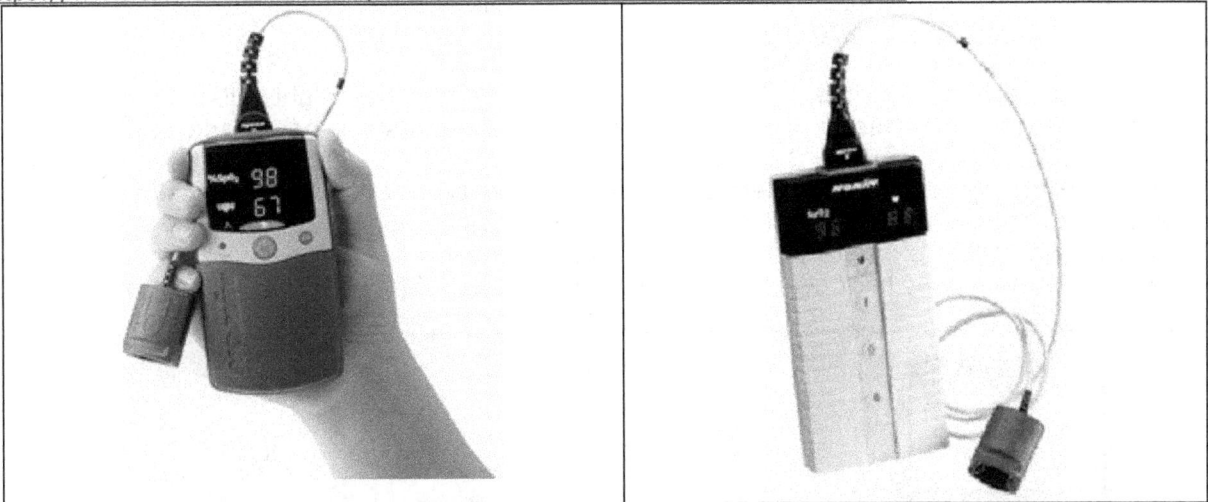

Courtesy of Nonin Medical, Inc.

Figure 2. 13 Nonin Pulse Oximeters can be used to do the "overnight pulse oximetry test."

+++

Concord Health Supply

9052 Terminal Avenue

Skokie, IL 60077, USA

Toll Free: 1-888.970.2999

Email: customerservice@concordhealthsupply.com

https://www.concordhealthsupply.com/

https://www.concordhealthsupply.com/Wrist-Pulse-Oximeters-s/46.htm

+++

Pulseoximeter.org

1616 Barclay Boulevard

Buffalo Grove IL, 60089

Phone: 847-234-0754

Email: info@pulseoximeter.org

https://www.pulseoximeter.org/

https://www.pulseoximeter.org/fingertip.html

+++

++

Southeastern Medical Supply
2711 Alpine Road, Ste. 210
Columbia, SC 29223, USA
Phone: 1-803-233-3691
Email: sales@semedicalsupply.com
http://www.semedicalsupply.com
https://www.semedicalsupply.com/Pulse-Oximeters-Pulse-Ox-Fingertip-Oximeter-s/48.htm

++

LOOKEE TECH

99 Wall Street #1698
New York, NY 10005
Phone: 1-818-287-7958
Email: Support@LookeeTech.com
https://www.lookeetech.com/
https://www.lookeetech.com/collections/fingertip-pulse-oximeters

♦ They have several pulse oximeters that can be used to do the "overnight pulse oximetry test." The results incluse AHI, Desaturation Index (number of events per hour) and SpO2 chart. AHI = Drops Per Hour, Oxygen Desaturatio Index (ODI) = Drops Over 4%.♦ They also have spot check oximeters, O2 Ring Oximeters, and many other types of finger pulse oximeters that can be used to do the "overnight pulse oximetry test" for sleep apnea.

♦ They are also selling oximeters on Amazon.com & Amazon.ca.

♦ They offer 30-day money back guaranty, and 1-year manufacturer's warranty on their oximeters.

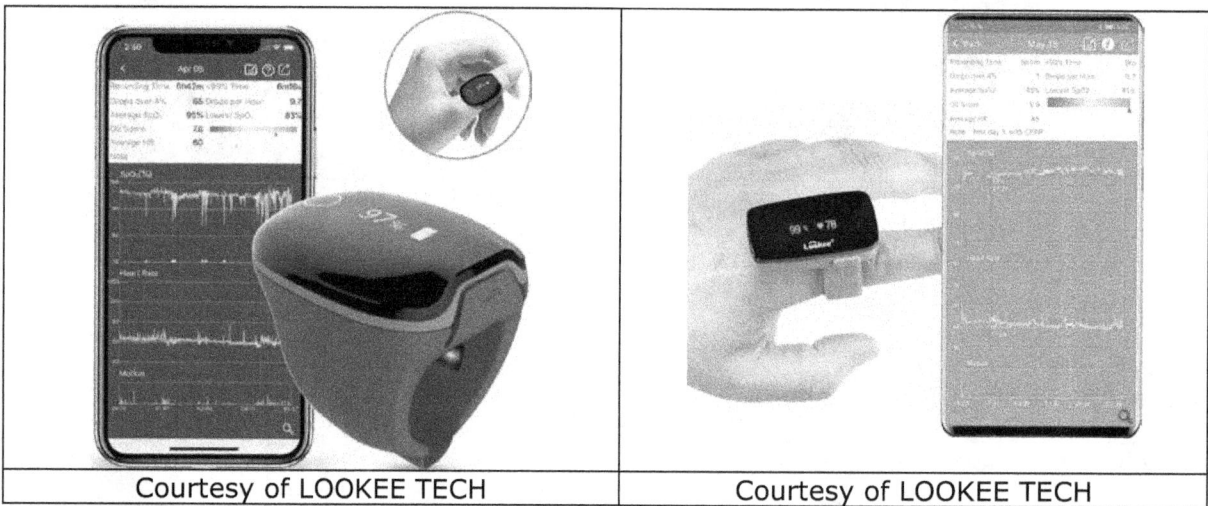

| Courtesy of LOOKEE TECH | Courtesy of LOOKEE TECH |

Figure 2.14 O2 Ring Oximeters can be used to do the "overnight pulse oximetry test."

++

++
EchoStore.com
Lake Bluff, IL, 60044, USA
Fax # 1-866-929-7118
Email: service@echostore.com
https://www.echostore.com/
https://www.echostore.com/healthcare.html
http://www.echostore.com/wrist-pulse-oximeter-cms-50f.html

♦ They have Wrist Pulse Oximeters, spot check oximeters, and they also have many other types of finger pulse oximeters that can be used to do the "overnight pulse oximetry test" for sleep apnea.
♦ They offer 30-day money bach guarantee and 1-year manufacturer's warranty on their oximeters.

++
VIATECH PULSE OXIMETERS
4E, Plant Building, Tingwei Industrial Park, No.6,
Liufang Road, Baoan District,
Shenzhen, Guangdong, China 518101
Email: Marketing@viatomtech.com   Phone (in China): +0086-755-86721161
https://www.viatomtech.com/ | https://www.viatomtech.com/pulse-oximeter

♦ They are the distributors of O2 Ring Oximeters. They have a variety of O2 Ring Oximeters. They can be used to do the "overnight pulse oximetry test" and final test results include Oxygen Desaturation Index, Minimum SpO2, Mean SpO2, Maximum SpO2, and SpO2 Chart.

++
WELLUE OXIMETERS
4E,3#,TingWei Park, Hong Lang North 2nd Road,
Bao'an District, Shenzhen, China
Email: support@getwellue.com   Phone (in China): +86-755 86638929
https://getwellue.com/collections/wellue

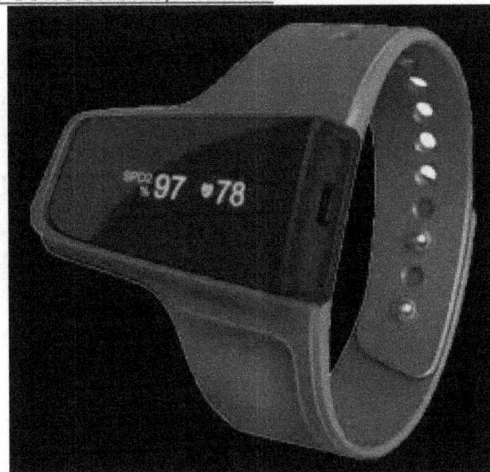

Courtesy of Wellue
Figure 2. 15 Wellue Wristwatch Oximeters can be used to do the "overnight pulse oximetry test."

♦ They are also located in China. They are selling oximeters and CPAP machines on Amazon.com & Amazon.ca.

♦ They have a variety of O2 Ring Oximeters. Wristwatch type oximeters that can be used to do the "overnight pulse oximetry test" for sleep apnea, and final test results include Oxygen Desaturation Index, Minimum SpO2, Mean SpO2, Maximum SpO2, and SpO2 Chart.

♦ They offer 30-day money back guaranty, and 1-year manufacturer's warranty on their oximeters.

++

SOME IMPORTANT TIPS

● Try to understand the difference between Spot Check Oximeter and the Oximeter for Continuous Monitoring. Remember that Spot Check Oximeters cannot be used to do the "overnight pulse oximetry test." Talk to the vendors, and purchase a pulse oximeter that can be used for continuous monitoring. Make sure it comes with software.

● Whenever you purchase an oximeter, test it by comparing the test result (Desaturation Index) with that of a high-precision Philips Respironics Pulse Oximeter or Nonin Pulse Oximeter by sleeping with both oximeters at the same time. If the oximeter you purchased is generating an error more than 10%, that means it is defective. Do not use such defective oximeter. Return that defective oximeter and get your money back within 30 days.

● **BE PREPARED TO FIGHT WITH DISHONENT RESELLERS:** Whenever you purchase an oximeter with 30-day money back guarantee, document the serial number of that oximeter. Ask the Reseller to email you the serial number of that oximeter you purchased. Let there be a witness (a friend or a family member) who knows the serial number of the device you purchased. Some resellers might falsely accuse you by saying that you returned a junk and dirty oximeter that was already broken and that was not the one they actually sold to you, and could refuse to refund your money. So be prepared to face and defend that kind of dishonest resellers. Always use a credit card to purchase the oximeter so that you can file a dispute with your credit card company if the oximeter is defective.

● **FINAL TIP:** <u>If it is too difficult for you to find a reliable oximeter on the market, or if you find that it is too expensive to purchase and own an oximeter for continuous monitoring, then you better borrow a high-precision oximeter (Philips Respironics Pulse Oximeter, Nonin Pulse Oximeter, or ResMed ApneaLink Air Device) from a sleep clinic or from a CPAP vendor once every 3 months or every 6 months, or as frequently as possible, and do the "overnight pulse oximetry text" at home. Maintain a journal and keep a record of all test results carefully, and take appropriate action to lower your Desaturation Index (events/hr). Please be noted that by lowering the Desaturation Index (events/hr), you can heal, cure, or even reverse your obstructive sleep apnea. Remember that it is possible to fully reverse obstructive sleep apnea by losing your excess body weight (there is scientific proof).</u>

++

VISITING A SLEEP APNEA SPECIALIST, MD

If you have been experiencing loud snoring, afternoon sleepiness with lack of energy throughout the day, and/or if you caught yourself falling asleep on the wheel while driving, your doctor would refer you to a sleep specialist who usually works in a hospital's sleep laboratory. When you visit the sleep specialist, after listening to the symptoms you describe, more specifically the snoring and afternoon sleepiness, and after understanding your overall health history and your parents' health history, the sleep specialist would first do the following physical examination.

PHYSICAL EXAMINATION

(i) Your doctor (a sleep specialist) would check your mouth and the inside of your throat to find out if an extra or large tissues are unusually hanging in your throat, and if they have been blocking the upper airway in your throat. Your doctor would also check if you have enlarged tonsils, an elongated uvula or a large tongue.

(ii) Your doctor would also check your nose to check for any sinuses and nasal congestion.

(iii) Your doctor would also monitor your naked body weight and your height, and might calculate your Body Mass Index (BMI) to understand if your weight is normal or if you are overweight or obese.

(iv) Your doctor would also measure your neck circumference and find out if your neck size is normal or not.

(v) Your doctor would also check your SpO2 level (percentage saturation of oxygen in the blood) using a spot check pulse oximeter, and find out if it is normal or not.

(vi) Your doctor would also check your heart rate and your blood pressure several times to understand if your sleep disorder has been causing the hypertension or high blood pressure.

(vii) Your doctor might also order some blood tests (fasting glucose, hemoglobin a1c, total cholesterol, LDL cholesterol, HDL cholesterol and several other tests) to find out if your sleep disorder has caused any further risks such as diabetes and heart disease, stroke, depression and other disorders.

(viii) Your doctor would also ask you if you smoke or drink alcohol often, and if your answer is yes, he/she would advise you to quit smoking and stop drinking alcohol.

(ix) Your doctor would also ask you repeatedly if your parents and/or siblings have any medical history of sleep apnea, insomnia or any other sleep-related problems to find out if your sleep disorder is hereditary or not. If any of your family members have the sleep disorder, you are likely to have it.

In order to understand the exact condition of your sleep disorder, and to properly diagnose you, your doctor will order the following tests:

a. **An overnight pulse oximetry test** to be performed by the patient at home to determine the Desaturation Index (number of sleep apnea events per hour). From this test, the severity of the sleep apnea condition (whether it is mild, moderate or severe) can be determined. This test also reports the values of minimum SpO2, mean SpO2 and maximum SpO2.

b. **An overnight polysomnogram test** which is organised in a hospital, and you may have to go back to that hospital to undergo this test with a sleep lab technician on a scheduled date.

POLYSOMNOGRAM TEST FOR SLEEP APNEA [46]

When you arrive at the sleep lab to undergo the polysomnogram test, the technician would ask you to wait in a room until you will be called. After some time, the technician places sticky patches and sensors/electrodes on your scalp, face, chest, limbs and a finger, and then asks you to sleep. The technician would also place elastic belts on your chest and belly to monitor your chest movements, and the strength and duration of the inhaled and exhaled breaths. When you fall asleep, those sensors/electrodes would record your brain activity, eye movements, heart rate and rhythm, blood pressure, and the amount of oxygen in the blood. The thin and flexible wires connected to those sensors/electrodes would transmit the data to a computer in the central processing room. You would not feel any discomfort during sleep because all the wires connected to the sensors/electrodes are soft and flexible.
Please refer to the Polysomnogram Picture below, which has two parts: part A and part B. Part A (upper part): The patient lies on the bed with sensors/electrodes and wires attached to his/her body. Part B (lower part): The chart shows the polysomnogram recording (blood oxygen level versus time), breathing event versus time and rapid eye movement (REM) versus time.

In some hospitals, when the polysmnogram study was about to be completed, the technician would hook a CPAP (Continuous Positive Airway Pressure) machine on you and a nasal mask so that you could breathe the air from the CPAP hose at low pressure, which would keep the airway fully open in your throat. The CPAP machine would monitor and record your SpO2, your pulse rate, the apneas and hypopneas & AHI when you sleep. The next morning, after the test the technician removes all the sensors and patches from your body and would instruct you to go home. The report will be sent to the doctor. The doctor would discuss the results with you during your next appointment with him.

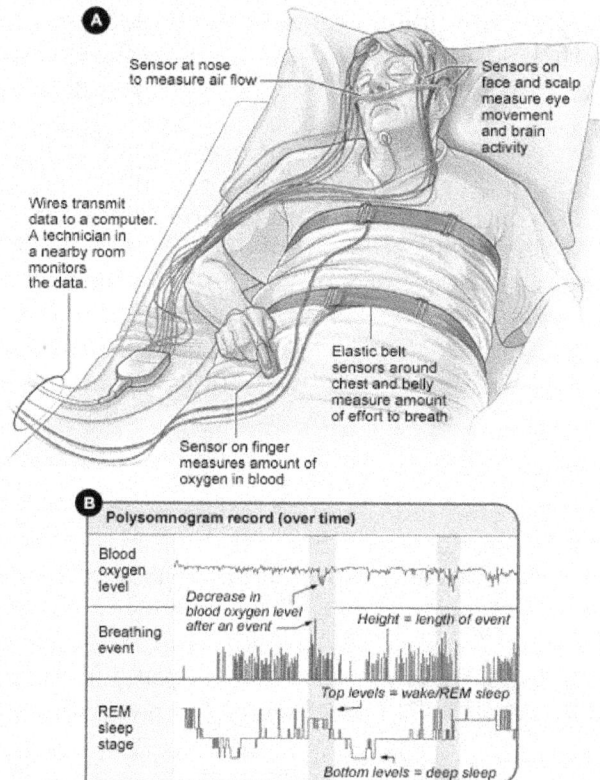

Source: FixYourSleep (Permission granted to reproduce the picture) [47]
Figure 2.16 A patient undergoing polysomnogram test in a local hospital.

IS A POLYSOMNOGRAM TEST NECESSARY?
POLYSOMNOGRAM TEST IS PROBLEMATIC AND UNNECESSARY.
HOME-BASED OVERNIGHT PULSE OXYMETRY TEST WOULD DO THE JOB.

● TOO MUCH NOISE AND BRIGHT LIGHTS IN THE SLEEP LAB COULD CAUSE INSOMNIA.
● The polysomnogram test should be conducted carefully in a very quiet and dark place so that the patient could fall asleep easily for at least 4 hours without being affected by any disturbance. But many hospitals do not organize the polysomnogram lab carefully to the full comfort of the patient because of the lack of funding.
● The sleep lab is not as comfortable and quiet as the patients expect. Hospitals try to accommodate several patients in one room by using dividers and by placing several beds side by side to do the polysomnogram test to multiple patients at the same time.
● Each patient is not completely isolated in a soundproof room and one patient could easily hear the noise from other patients. When the technician walks to a patient, all the other patients could hear the noise of his/her footsteps. When the technician talks to one patient, all the other patients could hear the noise and because of that noisy atmosphere, some patients may not be able to fall asleep, and thus not be able to complete the polysomnogram test successfully.
● If there is a noisy air conditioner in the sleep room, the patient may not be able to fall asleep. Or he/she may not be able to adjust to the room temperature as it could be too cold or too warm. Everyone prefers different temperatures.
● For every simple thing the patient needs, he/she needs to call the nurse by ringing the bell. The patient has no freedom to do anything, not even to pass the urine, on his/her own. The patient may have to walk a long distance with his/her sensors attached, escorted by a nurse, to go to the bathroom.
● This kind of bureaucratic and irritating aspects of the hospital stay could anger and annoy the patient and could cause insomnia. More than that, the bright lights in the hospital environment could cause insomnia to some patients.
● If the patient does not sleep peacefully for at least 4 hours, the polysomnogram test would be marked "incomplete."

That is why it would be a lot better to do the test at the comfort of the patient's home by using the pulse oximeter to find out the severity of the obstructive sleep apnea. The overnight pulse oximeter test would give all the information and the important results necessary to take decisions on treating the patient for obstructive sleep apnea.
All the patient has to do is: just learn how to use the pulse oximeter at home. Many CPAP vendors lend the pulse oximeter for free and teach the patient how to use it. Or the doctor's clinic in the hospital sleep lab also lend the pulse oximeter to their patients.

The patient could wear the pulse oximeter overnight or several nights, and then take it back to the CPAP vendor or the hospital clinic from where it was borrowed. They would upload the data from the pulse oximeter to the computer, and print out the results such as:
    a. The Desaturation Index (number of desaturation events/hr),
    b. Mean SpO2, Lowest SpO2 and Highest SpO2, SpO2 Vs Time Chart, Pulse Rate Vs Time Chart.

♦ From these results, it is possible to know the severity of the obstructive sleep apnea.
♦ Or the patient can purchase the pulse oximeter on the Internet, and can use it to monitor the sleep apnea progress every week or every month comfortably at home.
♦ Even though the polysomnogram test is more accurate, it is unnecessary to undergo the tedious test in a sleep lab because the hospital environment is not comfortable for the patient to sleep well.
♦ However a home-based "overnight pulse oximetry test" would do the job.

HOW TO KNOW IF SOMEONE HAS SLEEP APNEA OR NOT?

⊙ Take the "overnight pulse oximetry test" at home using a finger pulse oximeter for continuous monitoring (not the spot check oximeter).

⊙ Early in the morning, when you wake up after completing the test, upload the data from your pulse oximeter to your computer. The software will display a sleep apnea report on your computer monitor with the following results:

- ◆ Oxygen Desaturation Index (number of desaturation events/hr),
- ◆ Minimum SpO2, Mean SpO2 and Maximum SpO2,
- ◆ SpO2 Vs Time Chart, and Pulse Rate Vs Time Chart.

⊙ If your Oxygen Desaturation Index is 5 or more than 5 (but less than 15), that means you have mild sleep apnea.
⊙ If your Oxygen Desaturation Index is between 15 and 29, that means, you have moderate sleep apnea.
⊙ If your Oxygen Desaturation Index is is 30 or more than 30, that means you have secere sleep apnea (severe sleep apnea is extremely dangerous, so take action immediately).

Please refer to Table 2.8 (show below again for your convenience):

Table 2.8 Assessment guidelines of sleep apnea using desaturation index.

SpO2 Level (%)	Desaturation Index (Events/hr)	Assessment
96% - 99%	0 - 4	Normal
90% - 95%	5 - 14	Mild Sleep Apnea
80% - 90%	15 - 29	Moderate Sleep Apnea
< 80%	≥ 30	Severe Sleep Apnea

CHAPTER 2
REFERENCES

SNORING AND SLEEP APNEA

SNORING EXPLAINED
1. Snoring, Authored by Dr Oliver Starr, 18 Oct 2017.
https://patient.info/health/snoring-leaflet

2. Sleep Apnea and Snoring: What's the Difference? by Ruben Cohen, D.D.S.
https://www.huffingtonpost.com/ruben-cohen-dds/sleep-apnea-snoring_b_859974.html

3. The difference between loud snoring and obstructive sleep apnea by Robert Thomas.
https://www.snoringmouthpieceguide.com/the-difference-between-loud-snoring-and-obstructive-sleep-apnea/

4. What is the difference between snoring and sleep apnea? by Schellnoble Dentistry.
http://schellnoble.com/what-is-the-difference-between-snoring-and-sleep-apnea/

SLEEP APNEA EXPLAINED
5. Obstructive Sleep Apnea (from Wikipedia).
https://en.wikipedia.org/wiki/Obstructive_sleep_apnea

6. Sleep Apnea Picture (pharynx/trachea/windpipe).
https://www.google.ca/search?q=windpipe+pharynx&biw=1280&bih=890&tbm=isch&tbo=u&source=univ&sa=X&ved=0ahUKEwie5KCQjr7SAhUJ2GMKHROZAeIQsAQIKw#imgrc=T8EHZUTdJZ8o5M

7. Sleep Apnea, National Heart, Lung and Blood Institute.
https://www.nhlbi.nih.gov/health/health-topics/topics/sleepapnea

TYPES OF SLEEP APNEA
8. The different types of sleep apnea: Obstructive, Central and Mixed by Tamara Kaye Sellman RPSGT CCSH, Sleep Resolutions, March 7, 2017.
https://www.sleepresolutions.com/blog/the-different-kinds-of-sleep-apnea-obstructive-central-mixed

9. The 3 Types of Sleep Apnea Explained: Obstructive, Central & Mixed, Posted by Kevin Phillips, Alaska Sleep Education Center.
http://www.alaskasleep.com/blog/types-of-sleep-apnea-explained-obstructive-central-mixed

10. Falling Asleep.
http://fallingasleep.net/sleep-disorders/apnea

SYMPTOMS OF SLEEP APNEA, CAUSES OF SLEEP APNEA
RISK FACTORS, SIDE EFFECTS AND COMPLICATIONS
11. Being Alert to Sleep Apnea (Link between Sleep Apnea and Obesity) by Dr. Deepak Chopra, Posted on March 12, 2012.
http://www.huffingtonpost.com/deepak-chopra/sleep-apnea_b_1191695.html
https://www.deepakchopra.com/

12. Being Alert to Sleep Apnea (Snoring Explained) by Deepak Chopra™, M.D., Posted on January 07, 2012.
http://www.chopra.com/articles/being-alert-to-sleep-apnea#sm.0000oer4l81drecp9vy7y9zq6i1z2

13. 10 Signs and Symptoms of Sleep Apnea.
https://rmhealthy.com/10-signs-symptoms-sleep-apnea/

14. Obstructive Sleep Apnea: Symptoms, Causes, Treatments and Natural Remedies by an Unknown Author, Sleep-Apnea-Guide.com, 2020.
https://www.sleep-apnea-guide.com/obstructive-sleep-apnea.html

15. Obstructive and Central Sleep Apnea Causes by an Unknown Author, Sleep-Apnea-Guide.com, 2020.
https://www.sleep-apnea-guide.com/causes-of-sleep-apnea.html

16. Obstructive Sleep Apnea by Mayo Clinic Staff, Mayo Clinic, 2021
https://www.mayoclinic.org/diseases-conditions/obstructive-sleep-apnea/symptoms-causes/syc-20352090

17. Mayo Clinic Q and A: Neck size one risk factor for obstructive sleep apnea by Liza Torborg, Posted on June 20, 2015.
https://newsnetwork.mayoclinic.org/discussion/mayo-clinic-q-and-a-neck-size-one-risk-factor-for-obstructive-sleep-apnea/#:~:text=ANSWER%3A%20Having%20a%20neck%20circumference,block%20airflow%20as%20you%20sleep.

18. Obstructive Sleep Apnea (OSA) by WebMed, 2021.
https://www.webmd.com/sleep-disorders/sleep-apnea/understanding-obstructive-sleep-apnea-syndrome

19. Sleep Apnea by Cleveland Clinic Staff, Last reviewed by a Cleveland Clinic medical professional on March 03, 2020.
https://my.clevelandclinic.org/health/diseases/8718-sleep-apnea

20. Obstructive sleep apnea in adults by Mount Sinai Health Library, 2021.
https://www.mountsinai.org/health-library/diseases-conditions/obstructive-sleep-apnea-adults

21. Sleep Apnea: What it is, its risk factors, its health impacts, and how it can be treated, Written by Eric Suni, Medically Reviewed by Joel Gould, Sleepfoundation.org, Updated July 9, 2021.
https://www.sleepfoundation.org/sleep-apnea

22. Obstructive sleep apnea: Overview, National Center for Biotechnology Information (NCBI), U.S. National Library of Medicine, 8600 Rockville Pike, Bethesda, MD, 20894, USA, Created on July 22, 2011, Last Update on January 2, 2019.
https://www.ncbi.nlm.nih.gov/books/NBK279274/

23. Side Effects of Sleep Apnea.
http://www.istockphoto.com/ca/photo/sife-effects-from-sleep-apnea-gm512156549-46800846?st=_p_sleep%20apnea

24. Complications of Sleep Apnea.
http://www.istockphoto.com/ca/photo/complications-of-sleep-apnea-gm509367629-45852800

25. Complications of Obesity.
http://www.istockphoto.com/ca/photo/complications-of-obesity-gm535912311-57371134

SLEEP APNEA VERSUS COPD

26. What is the link between COPD and obstructive sleep apnea?, Written by Jon Johnson, medically reviewed by Raj Dasgupta, MD, Medical News Today, Posted on July 23, 2021.
https://www.medicalnewstoday.com/articles/copd-and-sleep-apnea

27. How is COPD Diagnosed? by COPD Foundation.
https://www.copdfoundation.org/What-is-COPD/Understanding-COPD/How-is-COPD-Diagnosed.aspx

28. A Deadly Duo: When COPD and OSA Overlap by Bill Pruitt, MBA, RRT, CPFT, AE-C, FAARC, RT Magazine Staff, Posted on May 9, 2014.
http://www.rtmagazine.com/2014/05/deadly-duo-copd-and-osa-overlap/

29. Sleep Apnea and COPD: What You Should Know, Written by Xavier Soler, MD, PhD, Posted on July 15, 2015.
https://www.copdfoundation.org/COPD360social/Community/COPD-Digest/Article/66/Sleep-Apnea-and-COPD-What-You-Should-Know.aspx

30. COPD: Facts, Statistics and You, Written by Jen Thomas, Medically reviewed by Debra Sullivan, Ph.D., MSN, R.N., CNE, COI, Updated and Posted on July 2, 2020.
https://www.healthline.com/health/copd/facts-statistics-infographic#COPD-types-and-frequency

OXYGEN SATURATION IN THE BLOOD (SpO2).

31. Permanent Diabetes Control (book), Authored by Rao Konduru, MS, PhD, DSc, Reviewed and Endorsed by Dr. Marshall Dahl, MD, PhD, Faculty of Medicine, University of British Columbia, Canada, Page 75, First Published in 2003, Revised and Rewritten in 2021.
http://mydiabetescontrol.com/

32. What is oxygen saturation?
http://www.pulseox.info/pulseox/what2.htm

33. Meaning of Blood Oxygen Saturation (SpO2).
https://www.healthcare4home.com/spo2-meaning/p.html

34. TORONTEX-E400 SPOT CHECK OXIMETER from 123CKECKUP.
https://123checkup.com/product/pulse-oximeter-torontek-e400w/

35. Oximetry by Medicinenet, Medical Author: George Schiffman, MD, FCCP, Medical Editor: Melissa Conrad Stöppler, MD.
http://www.medicinenet.com/oximetry/article.htm

36. Using the Pulse Oximeter, Manual Published by World Health Organization.
http://www.who.int/patientsafety/safesurgery/pulse_oximetry/who_ps_pulse_oxymetry_tutorial2_advanced_en.pdf

37. What is the oxygen desaturation index (ODI) measured on a sleep study?
What Is the Meaning of the Sleep Study AHI in Adults with Sleep Apnea?
By Brandon Peters, MD - Reviewed by a board-certified physician, Updated May 30, 2016.
https://www.verywell.com/oxygen-desaturation-index-3015362

38. Apnea Hypopnea Index (AHI): Understanding the Obstructive Sleep Apnea Results by Harvard Medical School.
http://healthysleep.med.harvard.edu/sleep-apnea/diagnosing-osa/understanding-results

FINGER PULSE OXIMETERS

39. Philips Respironics 920M Handheld Pulse Oximeter by Philips.com.
http://www.usa.philips.com/healthcare/product/HC920MP/920m-plus-handheld-oximeter

40. Nonin-8500 Handheld Pulse Oximeter by Nonin.com.
https://www.nonin.com/products/8500/

ResMed ApneaLink™ Air Home Sleep Testing Device

41. ResMed ApneaLink™ Air" Diagnostic Device for Sleep Apnea by ResMed.
https://www.resmed.com/en-us/healthcare-professional/products-and-support/home-sleep-testing/apnealink-air/

42. Patient Instructions, ResMed ApneaLink™ Air" Diagnostic Device for Sleep Apnea by ResMed.
https://document.resmed.com/documents/products/diagnostic/apnealink-air/patient-instructions/228691_apnealink-air_patient-instructions_glo_eng.pdf

43. Clinical Guide, ResMed ApneaLink™ Air" Diagnostic Device for Sleep Apnea by ResMed.
https://airview.resmed.com/resources/welcome-page/pdf/Apnealink-Air_clinical_guide_glo_eng.pdf

44. YouTube Video: How to use the ResMed ApneaLink™ Air Home Sleep Testing Device by ResMed.
https://www.youtube.com/watch?v=awa4z2fFn7A
https://www.youtube.com/watch?v=UEdGJp5fL40

45. Take-Home Sleep Apnea Test Instructions (There is a ResMed video on this page) by SLEEPSOMATICS DIAGNOSIC CENTER, 2211 W PARMER LN, AUSTIN, TX, 78727, USA.
https://www.sleepsomatics.com/sleepsomatics-journal-blog-about-sleep/take-home-sleep-apnea-test-instructions/2016/10/13

POLYSOMNOGRAM TEST IN A SLEEP LAB

46. How is Sleep Apnea Diagnosed by National Heart, Lung and Blood Institute.
http://www.nhlbi.nih.gov/health/health-topics/topics/slpst/during
https://www.nhlbi.nih.gov/health/health-topics/topics/sleepapnea/diagnosis

47. Source: Fix Your Sleep Today, What Can I Expect from A Sleep Study?
Permission granted to reproduce the polysomnogram picture.
http://fixyoursleeptoday.com/what-to-expect-from-a-sleep-study

CHAPTER 3   SLEEP APNEA TREATMENT Section-I

⬤ THE CPAP THERAPY
⬤ THE CPAP MACHINES
⬤ THE CPAP MASKS

TABLE OF CONTENTS

CHAPTER 3   SLEEP APNEA TREATMENT Section-I
THE CPAP THERAPY & THE CPAP MACHINE

WHAT IS THE CPAP THERAPY?

● **CPAP means "Continuous Positive Airway Pressure,"** which further means that the CPAP machine pumps air into your throat, and helps maintain continuous, positive, very low and comfortable air pressure in the airway of your throat, keeps the airway open all the time, and stops snoring whenever you sleep with it. The CPAP machine has a mini compressor in it, which blows air into the mouth and/or nose at a very low and comfortable pressure, and keeps the airway always open by preventing the soft tissue of the throat muscles from collapsing onto the airway, thereby unblocking, abolishing snoring, shallow breathing and oxygen desaturation events. As long as you wear the CPAP machine during the night while sleeping, the CPAP machine kills most apneas and hypopneas, and keeps your AHI (Apnea Hypopnea Index) perfectly normal, under 5. As the airway remains always open, sufficient amount of air passes into the lungs freely, and maintains normal blood oxygen level (SpO2 = 96% to 99%) all the time during sleep. You wake up in the morning fully satisfied with your sleep and completely refreshed. You would not experience any symptoms of obstructive sleep apnea such as tiredness, low energy or lack of breath when you wake up in the morning.

● As you sleep all the night with perfectly normal SpO2 levels, your overall health improves. If you take appropriate steps to lose your excess body weight, your obstructive sleep apnea will be progressively healed and even reversed.

● CPAP was first invented by an "Australian Professor Colin Sullivan" in 1980 when he was a Senior Lecturer in Medicine at the University of Sydney, and Honorary Physician at the Royal Prince Alfred Hospital. Continuous positive airway pressure (CPAP) has since become "gold standard" treatment for patients with obstructive sleep apnea all over the world. [1, 2, 3]

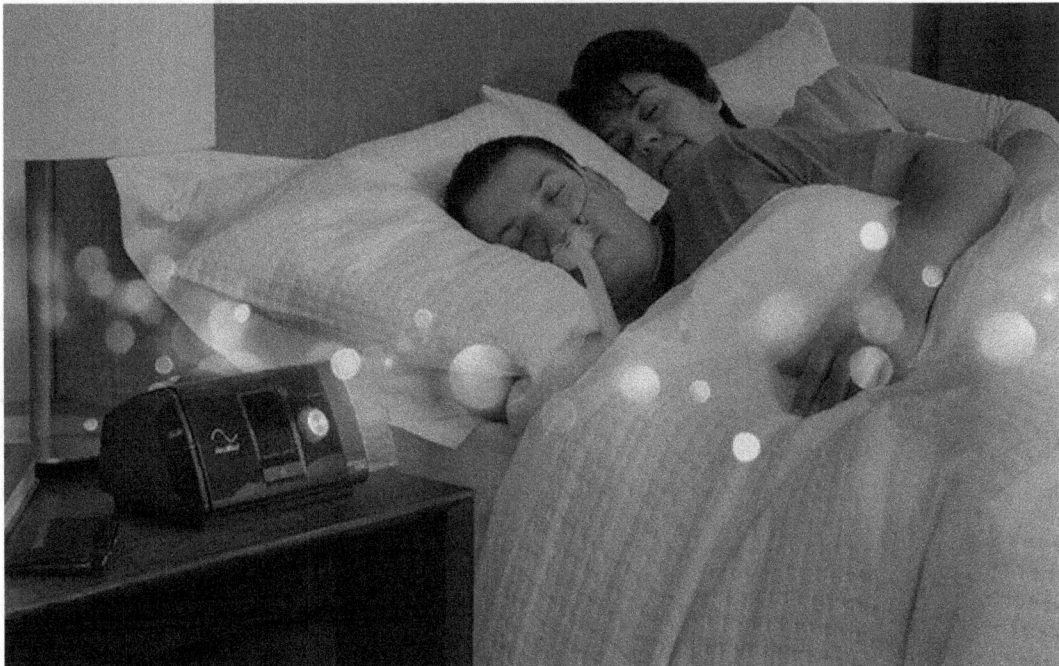

Courtesy of ResMed
Figure 3.1 A sleep apnea patient is sleeping with the ResMed CPAP machine.

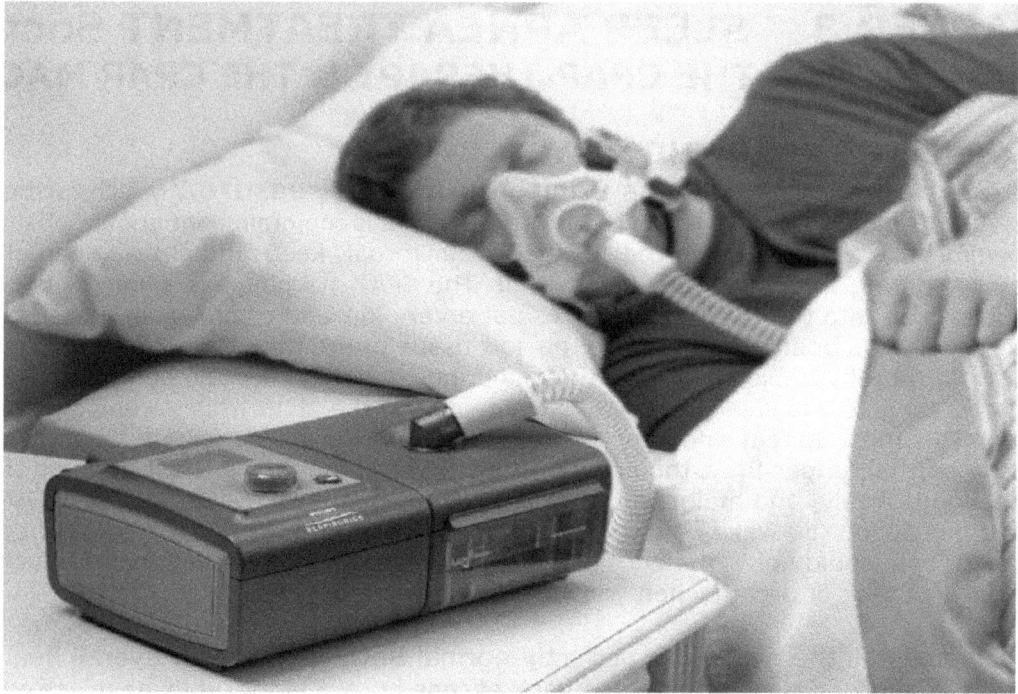

Courtesy of Philips Respironics
Figure 3.2 A sleep apnea patient is sleeping with the Respironics CPAP machine.

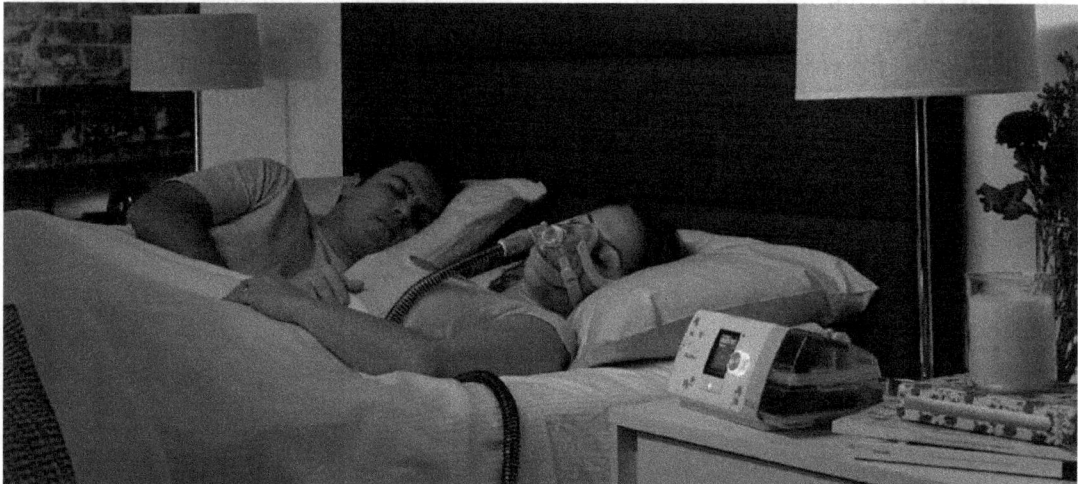

Courtesy of ResMed
Figure 3.3 A sleep apnea patient is sleeping with the ResMed CPAP machine.

• The CPAP therapy and CPAP machine require a doctor's prescription (although some CPAP machines can be purchased online without any prescription). The CPAP machine is a medical device that supplies a gentle flow of positive pressured, filtered and humidified air creating an artificial splint allowing the airway in the throat to remain fully open.

• The CPAP's motor is a mini compressor that draws air in gently through an air-filter and then delivers into a humidifier. The humidifier should be filled with distilled water (never use tap water). The filtered and humidified air is then driven into a mask by means of a lightweight and flexible tubing. The air filter should be replaced once every month.

• Usually a nasal pillows mask is recommended because of its simplicity and comfort (you can use full-face mask if you are accustomed to it or if you are a mouth-breather). The nasal pillows mask has a very comfortable hose that goes into the nose via a gel pillow that seals the person's nostrils when inserted. The nasal pillow has a smooth and delicate cushion, available in three sizes: small, medium and large, so that a person could easily adapt to the mask and the air flow. The mask also has a headgear and straps so that a person can easily adjust them to the desired tightness to avoid leaks. A variety of CPAP machines and the masks are shown in the pictures below.

• The CPAP machine blows air at a very low pressure so that the airway/windpipe in the throat remains open and sufficient amount of air passes into the lungs. So the CPAP machine, as long as the mask is plugged into your nose and/or mouth, maintains normal SpO2 levels. That means as long you sleep with the CPAP machine, you are sleeping without sleep apnea and protecting yourself from the danger of low blood oxygen levels.

TYPES OF THE CPAP MACHINES

When a person experiences the symptoms of sleep apnea, the family physician refers him/her to a sleep specialist in a nearby sleep lab. After a thorough medical check-up, the certified sleep specialist orders an overnight pulse oximetry test to be performed at the patient's home, and/or polysomnogram test to be performed in a hospital. Based on the results obtained from the aforementioned tests, the doctor prescribes the CPAP therapy by using one of the following CPAP machines:

The CPAP therapy unquestionably the most successful treatment available to relieve obstructive sleep apnea. <u>The purpose of the CPAP therapy is to keep the AHI (Apnea Hypopnia Index) under 5 events per hour, and to keep the mean SpO2 level perfectly normal</u>. The CPAP machine does not monitor and record SpO2 level, but if the AHI is under 5 events per hour, the mean SpO2 would automatically be normal. Each person is different so each person has to research and try several types of CPAP machines (shown below) in achieving this goal. Generally a qualified sleep specialist, by looking into the pulse oximetry or polysmnogram tests results, determines which of the following machines would suit a particular patient, and prescribes the appropriate CPAP machine and the matching mask. However it is the patient's responsibility to check the "sleep report" every morning, and make sure that the AHI is under 5 events per hour.
(i) CPAP (Continuous Positive Airway Pressure) The machine delivers air at a fixed pre-set pressure throughout the sleep, and it is the older type of CPAP therapy many people have been using. CPAP suits and works for most people to treat obstructive sleep apnea at fixed pressure unless a patient develops specific breathing problems, and needs variable pressures. Most older machines are CPAPs.
(ii) APAP (Automatic Positive Airway Pressure) [5, 6] The APAP machine is a modified CPAP machine, and delivers air automatically at different pressures at different situations. It is capable to self-adjust the air pressure on breath-by-breath basis if need be. The machine senses when you fall asleep, and the air pressure ramps up from minimum to maximum so that your airway remains fully open and you will not snore. The APAP machine uses algorithms, which sense minute changes in your breathing then adjusts itself to provide the best pressure setting for your specific sleep apnea therapy requirements. Most newly released CPAPs are APAPs.

(iii) BiPAP (Bilivel Positive Airway Pressure), or [5, 7]
   VPAP (Variable Positive Airway Pressure)

BiPAP machines are mostly used in hospitals. When you breathe in, a BiPAP machine delivers more air pressure. This is also known as inspiratory positive airway pressure (IPAP). When you breathe out, the machine reduces the air pressure. This is called expiratory positive airway pressure (EPAP).

The difference between CPAP and BiPAP machines is based on how the air pressure is delivered to the mask. BiPAP machines deliver two levels of air pressure where as CPAP machines deliver a continuous level of fixed air pressure. CPAPs are typically the first treatment option for people with obstructive sleep apnea. The continuous pressure holds the airway in the throat open, and stops snoring, and there's no need for two different pressures. However the variable positive airway pressure offered by BiPAP machines is more comfortable and makes the therapy more enjoyable.

(iv) ASV (Adaptive Servoventilation Device) [8, 9]

ASV is used in hospitals for those people who suffer from complex sleep apnea (central apneas emerging with use of CPAP or bilevel PAP therapy).

ASV is similar to CPAP devices, but it is a newer technology. These devices track how you breathe while you sleep. They react to your breathing pattern and adjust air pressure to help you breathe more normally during the night. Your doctor will set the initial air pressure on your ASV. This "smart" machine has technology that allows it to change how much air pressure it gives you and how often to keep your airways open so you can breathe.

Whenever the ASV machine detects abnormalities in breathing, it intervenes with just enough support to maintain the patient's breathing at 90% of what had been normal for that patient prior to the abrupt change in breathing. When the patient's breathing problem ends, the machine re-adjusts itself to the patient's normal breathing pattern. When the patient's breathing is stable, ASV provides just enough pressure support to provide an approximate 50% reduction in the work of breathing for the patient, therefore making the therapy much more comfortable for the patient.

WONDERFUL HEALTH BENEFITS OF THE CPAP THERAPY

- The CPAP therapy is the best, most effective and enjoyable therapy if you know how to use the CPAP machine and the mask correctly. It promotes restful sleep, improves concentration and focus on daily activities throughout the day, enhances memory, and boosts daytime energy.
- The CPAP therapy has been found to be 100% effective in keeping normal SpO2 level (SpO2 = 96% to 99%), and in treating wide fluctuations of the SpO2 level in the sleep.
- Either apnea hypopnea index (AHI) or Oxygen Desaturation Index (ODI) can be maintained perfectly normal (under 5 desaturation events per hour) by means of the powerful CPAP therapy.
- Snoring can be completely abolished by means of the CPAP therapy by maintaining the appropriate air pressure in the mask trough which a person inhales air.
- The CPAP therapy is being used for patients of all ages to treat their sleep disorder problems, mostly moderate and severe obstructive sleep apnea.
- Of course the mild obstructive sleep apnea can also be one 100% effectively and very easily treated with the powerful CPAP therapy.

◆ The CPAP machine is designed with a humidifier inside so that the filtered air is humidified before passing through the airway, throat and lungs. The humidified air can case symptoms of a cold, sore throat or cough.

◆ The CPAP therapy is also being successfully used for children to treat respiratory distress syndrome or bronchopulmonary dysplasia. It can also be used in treating acute hypoxaemic respiratory failure in children [1]

◆ It was shown that the CPAP therapy can also be used to treat the Upper Airway Resistance Syndrome (UARS) as the condition progresses, in order to prevent it from developing into obstructive sleep apnea. [1]

◆ A meta-analysis showed that the CPAP therapy may reduce erectile dysfunction symptoms in male patients with obstructive sleep apnea. [1]

◆ In March 2020, the United States FDA suggested that CPAP devices may be used to support patients affected by COVID-19 if SpO2 level falls below normal. [1]

ADAPTING TO THE CPAP THERAPY WOULD BE AN UPHILL BATTLE!

◆ Adapting and getting accustomed to the CPAP therapy is a daunting and challenging task, as very many people with sleep apnea most commonly do not adhere to the recommended method of the CPAP therapy. Up to 50% of the people discontinue the use of the CPAP machine in the first year, and look for an oral appliance or mouthpiece because the CPAP therapy in the beginning stage requires a lot of patience, high self discipline and high willpower.

◆ Many therapists staffed by the CPAP vendors do not train their sleep apnea patients properly, leaving the patients in a dilemma of many confusions, questions and doubts on using the CPAP machine and mask, and in understanding the sleep apnea condition. They are there to sell CPAP machines at highly inflated prices. Even many sleep clinic doctors do not provide proper training to their patients on how to understand and use the CPAP machine and mask. Most sleep apnea patients purchase CPAP machine along with a mask from the local CPAP vendors, and after the purchase, they are on their own. They go home and start the therapy on their own without proper training. They become fed up by their noisy and leaky masks, and give up the CPAP therapy, and look for an oral appliance or mouthpiece instead. There is nobody to help them at home and answer their questions when they are annoyed by the complicated and leaky masks. They simply remove the mask while sleeping, and sleep without it. There could be very many cases like that.

SIDE EFFECTS OF THE CPAP THERAPY

◆ The non-invasive nature of the CPAP therapy makes it the "gold standard" form of treatment for obstructive sleep apnea. Many sleep apnea patients enjoy the CPAP therapy and live without any symptoms of sleep apnea, thanking the CPAP invention. However, for some people, the extra flow of humidified air from a malfunctioning humidifier, delivered at high air pressure from the CPAP machine to the mask, may cause dry mouth, dry tongue, dry nose, dry throat, runny nose, stuffy nose, nosebleeds, sneezing, nasal congestion, insomnia and other problems. However these problems can usually be addressed and minimized by adjusting the tube temperature of the humidifier, by wearing chinstraps, and by working closely with a knowledgeable and experienced therapist or sleep clinic doctor. [1, 3, 4]

◆ Some people experience difficulty adjusting to the CPAP therapy and report the general discomfort, nasal congestion, abdominal bloating, sensations of claustrophobia while adapting to the CPAP mask, mask leaks and associated noise, and feeling of inconvenience throughout the night. Many patients don't know how to exercise patience, high self-discipline and high willpower to handle the aforementioned problems, and eventually give up the CPAP therapy, and look for an alternative therapy (oral appliance or mouthpiece). [1]

DISADVANTAGES OF THE CPAP THERAPY

(i) <u>The CPAP therapy does not heal, cure or reverse obstructive sleep apnea. The CPAP therapy solely controls sleep apnea and keeps your blood oxygen level (SpO2 level) and the Oxygen Desaturation Index (events per hour) perfectly normal only during the time you use it.</u> Whenever the CPAP mask is on your nose and/or mouth, the air pressure keeps your airway open by preventing the soft tissue of the throat muscle from collapsing and blocking the airway, thereby keeping your blood oxygen level (SpO2 level) perfectly normal. But when you sleep without wearing the CPAP, the soft tissue in the throat muscle collapses and blocks the airway as usually, and you would be living with the symptoms of obstructive sleep apnea.

(ii) <u>The CPAP therapy is exactly like using eyeglasses for seeing and reading.</u> You would be able to see clearly and read clearly whenever you wear the eyeglasses, and you would not be able to see clearly and read clearly whenever you don't wear the eyeglasses. The eyeglasses do not cure your eyesight but help control your sight and help you see and read clearly only when you wear them. The CPAP machine works exactly like that. That is to say that the CPAP therapy does not cure your sleep apnea, but solely controls sleep apnea by keeping your SpO2 level and number of oxygen desaturation events normal only during the time you use it.

(iii) The patient may not feel comfortable wearing a mask while sleeping with his/her spouse or partner. It will take some time to get used to the CPAP therapy.

(iv) There could be air leaks in the mask and you wouldn't even know when sleeping if the machine is not working perfectly or not. There is no alarm system that would wake you up from your sleep after detecting a defective mask and/or broken machine.

(v) The CPAP manufacturing companies do not provide the essential and the most important technical support over the phone directly to the patients to resolve the technical problems developed while using the CPAP machine and mask. When the patients are not confident and highly knowledgeable in using and troubleshooting the CPAP machine and mask, they lose interest on the CPAP therapy, and many patients say "good bye" to the CPAP therapy.

PLEASE DO NOT GIVE UP THE CPAP THERAPY

● ALWAYS REMEMBER that the CPAP therapy is the best treatment for obstructive sleep apnea. No matter how severe your sleep apnea is, whether it is mild, moderate or severe, you can protect yourself from the unbearable and yet dangerous symptoms of the obstructive sleep apnea, and can live like a normal person by means of the CPAP therapy. There is no other therapy that comes even close to the CPAP therapy to treat obstructive sleep apnea.

● Most importantly, the CPAP therapy maintains your SpO2 level and the Oxygen Desaturation Index (events per hour) perfectly normal throughout the night as long as the CPAP machine is working perfectly. There is no other therapy or mouthpiece that can do you such a wonder.

● Broken or defective CPAP machines look like working by blowing air into the mask but generate weird sleep report by the end of the night (some patients do not even notice it). You therefore must be vigilant, wise and knowledgeable, and should check it every day, and make sure that your CPAP machine is working perfectly and generating the sleep report that makes sense.

● <u>Never sleep without hooking up to the CPAP machine if you have sleep apnea.</u> Be patient and persistent, and please do not give up the CPAP therapy by being frustrated due to the complexity of using the CPAP machine. Learn how to use it with confidence. With diligence, patience, self-discipline and will power, you can get used to the CPAP therapy. This guide will teach you everything you need to get used to the CPAP therapy and to master the topic.

CPAP MACHINES [10]

"CPAP machine" is an electronic device that is used to treat and relieve sleep apnea. A CPAP machine has a mini motor inside and delivers air through tubing and into a mask to keep your airway open while you sleep. This process is known as sleep therapy or CPAP therapy and is designed to help you get a restful night's sleep. Most CPAP machines are being manufactured by ResMed, Respironics, Fisher & Paykel. A typical CPAP machine (ResMed CPAP machine) is comprised of the following 5 major components:

♦ A Built-In Device (ResMed AirSense 10 CPAP Machine)
♦ Power Cord with AC-DC Adapter
♦ ClimateLine Air Heated Tube (Hose)
♦ Humidifier (Chamber), Air Filters, and
♦ Laptop Style Travel Bag

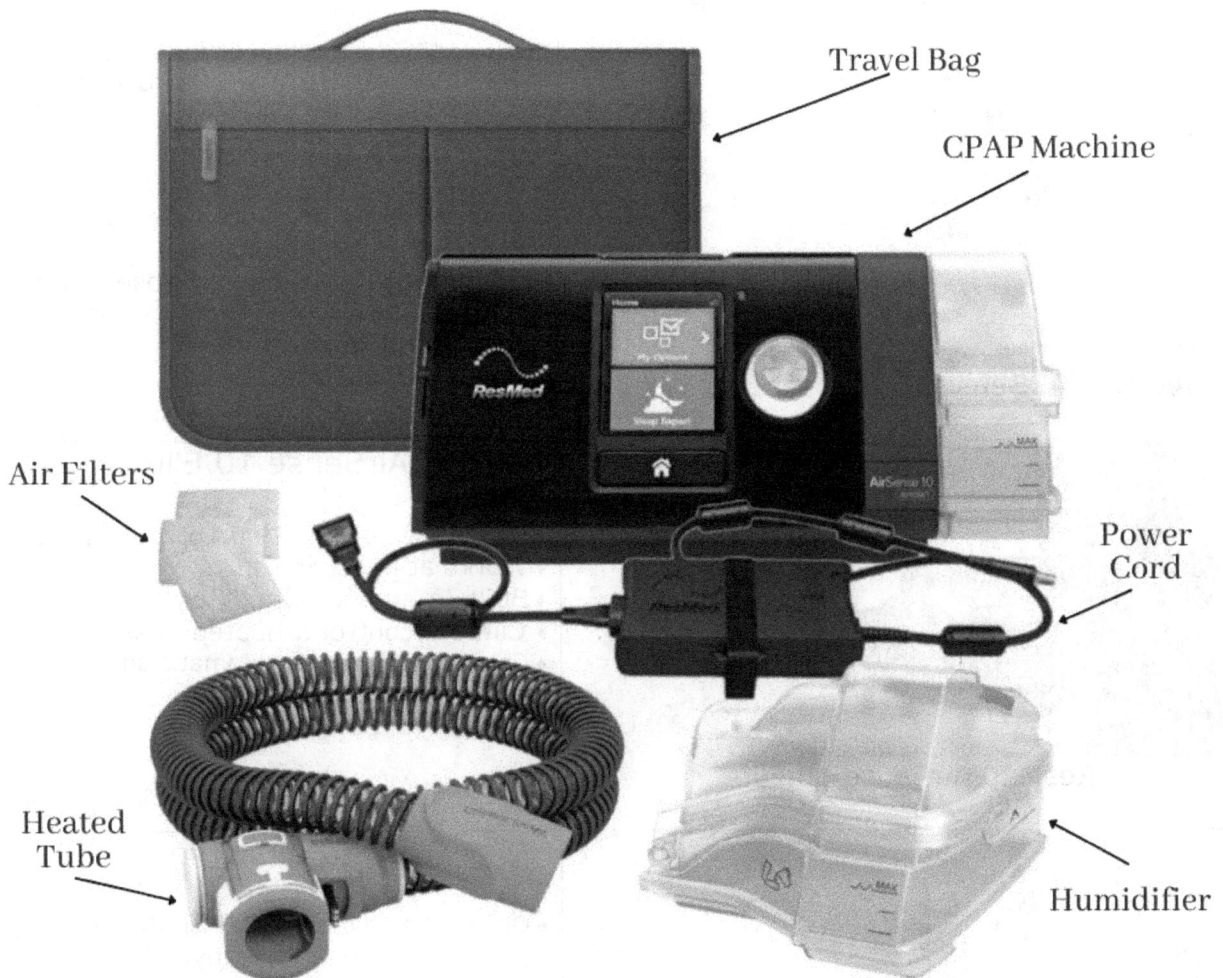

Courtesy of ResMed
Figure 3.4 The components of a typical CPAP machine.

Table 3.1 The list of ResMed CPAP machines, being used to control sleep apnea.

ResMed CPAP Machines [10, 11]	
ResMed CPAP machines are being used everywhere!	
ResMed AirSense 10 Autoset	**ResMed AirSense 10 Autoset** ♦ One of the quietest CPAPs on the market ♦ Delayed ramp pressure increase ♦ Built-In heated humidifier ♦ Climate control & heated hose (Tube) ♦ Color LCD display & automatic adjustment ♦ Although it is called CPAP, it has the features of APAP
ResMed AirSense 10 Autoset (For Her)	**ResMed AirSense 10 Autoset** [For Her Version] ♦ One of the quietest CPAPs on the market ♦ Delayed ramp pressure increase ♦ Built-In heated humidifier ♦ Climate control & heated hose (Tube) ♦ Color LCD display & automatic adjusting ♦ Although it is called CPAP, it has the features of APAP
ResMed AirSense 10 Elite	**ResMed AirSense 10 Elite** ♦ One of the quietest CPAPs on the market ♦ Works at fixed pressure ♦ Built-In heated humidifier ♦ Climate control & heated hose (Tube) ♦ Color LCD display & automatic adjusting ♦ Although it is called CPAP, it has the features of APAP
ResMed AirCurve 10	**ResMed AirCurve 10** ♦ One of the quietest CPAPs on the market ♦ Works for bileval therapy ♦ Built-In heated humidifier ♦ Climate control & heated hose (Tube) ♦ Color LCD display & automatic adjusting ♦ Although it is called CPAP, it has the features of APAP

ResMed AirCurve ASV

♦ One of the quietest CPAPs on the market
♦ Offers personalized therapy
♦ Works for ASV therapy
♦ Also works for Bilevel therapy
♦ Auto servo-ventilation
♦ Climate Control humidifier
♦ Vsync leak protection

ResMed AirCurve ASV

ResMed AirMini CPAP

AirMini is the world's smallest CPAP, weighing less than a pound and fitting in the palm of your hand.

♦ One of the quietest CPAPs on the market
♦ Works for bileval therapy
♦ works without humidification of air
♦ Color LCD display & automatic adjusting
♦ Although it is called CPAP, it has the features of APAP

ResMed AirMini

ResMed AirSense 11 Autoset

♦ The ResMed AirSense™ 11 AutoSet™ is a premium auto-adjusting pressure device with integrated heated humidifier, wireless connectivity, advanced event detection and patient support features.
♦ ResMed AirSense 11 is currently available only in the United States and is expected to be available in other countries (no Internet sales).

ResMed AirSense 11 Autoset
ResMed's most recent CPAP

Courtesy of ResMed!

Table 3.2 The list of Respironics CPAP machines, being used to control sleep apnea.

Respironics CPAP Machines [12]	
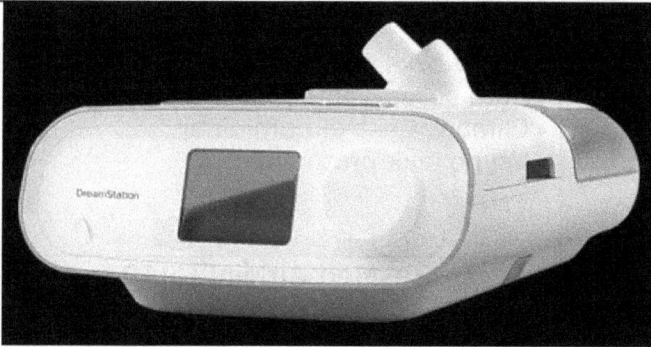 DreamStation CPAP and Bi-level Therapy Systems	**DreamStation CPAP and Bi-level Therapy Systems** ♦ Respirinics website claims that: DreamStation positive airway pressure (PAP) sleep therapy devices are designed to be as comfortable and easy to experience as sleep is intended to be. Connecting patients and care teams, DreamStation devices empower users to embrace their care with confidence, and enable care teams to practice efficient and effective patient management.
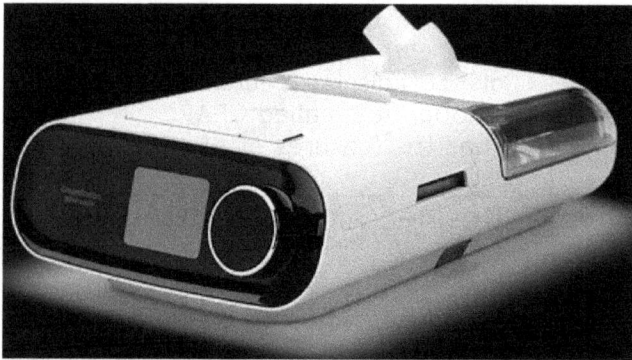 DreamStation BiPAP autoSV	**DreamStation BiPAP autoSV Servo-ventilation system** ♦ Respirinics website claims that: For patients with central sleep apnea, complex sleep apnea and periodic breathing, DreamStation BiPAP autoSV is designed to deliver optimal ventilation with minimal intervention. Its clinically proven algorithm provides support when needed, and works with patient breathing patterns to minimize applied pressure, pressure support and machine breaths - so sleep apnea patients can experience comfortable, restful sleep.
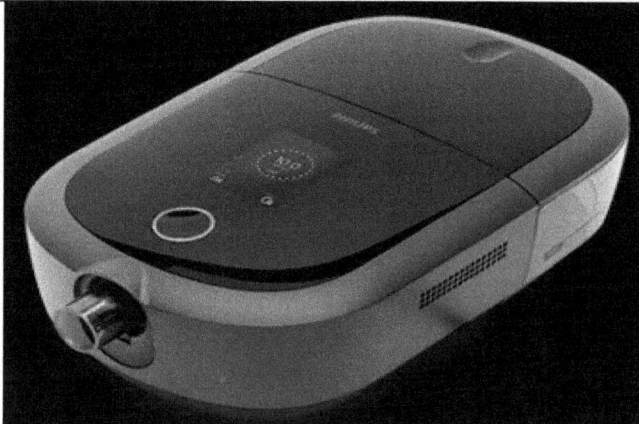 DreamStation 2 Auto CPAP Advanced	DreamStation 2 Auto CPAP Advanced ♦ Respirinics website claims that: DreamStation 2 Auto CPAP Advanced is the next evolution in clinically proven, integrated sleep solutions. It's designed to provide operational efficiencies and a simplified user experience, including flexible setup, a fully integrated humidifier and modem, advanced comfort features and patient management tools.
Courtesy of Philips Respironics!	

Table 3.3 The list of Fisher & Paykel CPAP machines, being used to control sleep apnea.

Fisher & Paykel CPAP Machines [13, 14]	
 SleepStyle AutoCPAP	**SleepStyle AutoCPAP** ♦ The website of Fisher & Paykel claims that: SleepStudy AutoCPAP is designed to make therapy comfortable and straightforward, the device features automatic treatment pressure adjustments, large and responsive buttons, and a dishwasher-safe humidifier chamber. This award-winning machine is easy to set-up and even easier to operate thanks to the user-friendly menu. Just press the start button, and your therapy will begin. Customers also appreciate the dishwasher-safe humidifier chamber, which is easy to fill and clean, and the simple menu navigation.
 F&P ICON™ NOVO F&P ICON™ PREMO	**F&P ICON™ NOVO and F&P ICON™ PREMO** ♦ The website of Fisher & Paykel claims that: Fisher and Paykel has modified their SleepStyle line of CPAP machines and combined those and more to enhance patient comfort and provide a personalized therapy system. The ICON Premo incorporates Optional ThermoSmart technology and advanced reporting into a streamlined body. The built-in heated humidifier and optional heated hose delivers condensation-free humidification at the touch of a button. The ICON is ideal for home or travel and comes with an alarm clock and Mp3 player as well as a hard protective case.
Courtesy of Fisher & Packel!	

Table 3.4 The list of ResMed CPAP masks, being used to control sleep apnea.

CPAP MASKS [10, 15]

A sleep apnea patient who is on CPAP therapy should research several masks, and select the one that perfectly suits to their face and the taste. Some people like and easily get accustomed to the full face masks. But many other people dislike full face masks by being claustrophobic, and prefer nasal pillows masks. In general nasal pillows masks are more comfortable and easily adaptable. A sleep apnea patient should also learn how to connect the mask and the the tube (hose) by means of a connector (swivel adapter), and how to adjust the straps on the nasal pillows mask so that there will not by any leaks while sleeping with the CPAP machine and mask.

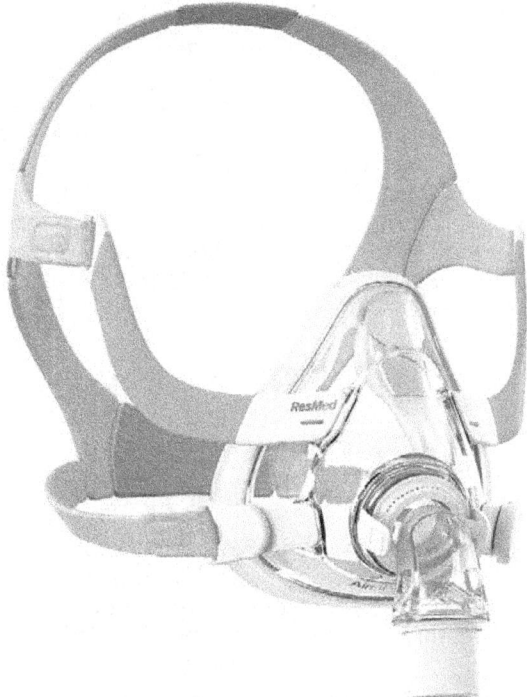
ResMed Air Fit F20 Full Face Mask

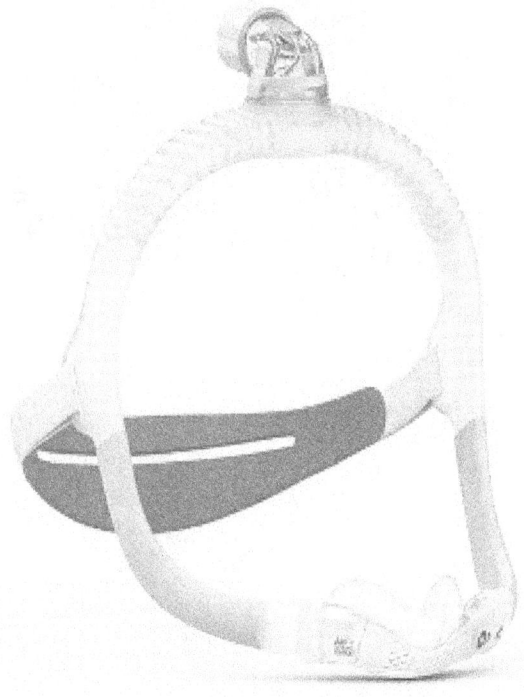
ResMed AirFit N30i Nasal Cradle Mask

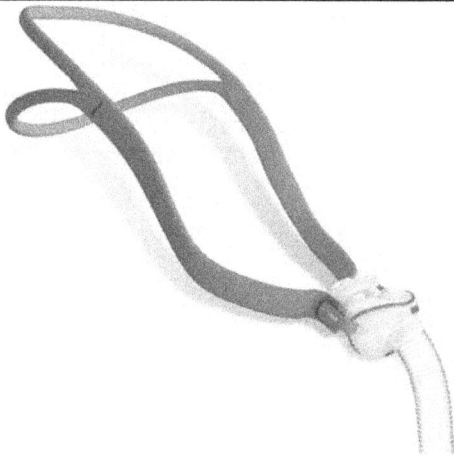
ResMed Air Fit P10 Nasal Pillow Mask

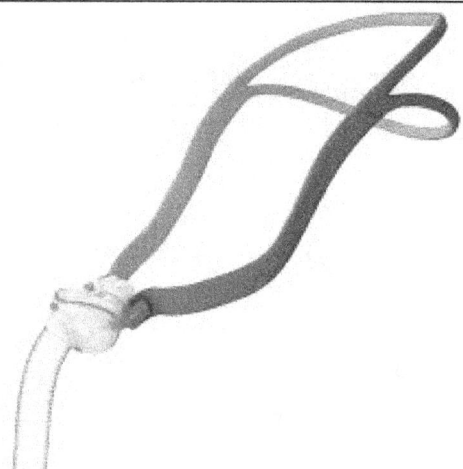
ResMed Air Fit P10 Nasal Pillow Mask (For Her)

Courtesy of ResMed!

PHILIPS RESPORONICS NUANCE PRO GEL NASAL PILLOW MASK [15, 16]

Phillps Respironics Nuance Pro Gel Nasal Pillow Mask is being used by many patients as is found to be confortable. The pillows perfectly seal the nostrils so that there will not be any air leaks, and pillow cushions are so soft that a patient can easily adapt to the mask. By adjusting the straps, it is possible to fit perfectly to any size of the face.

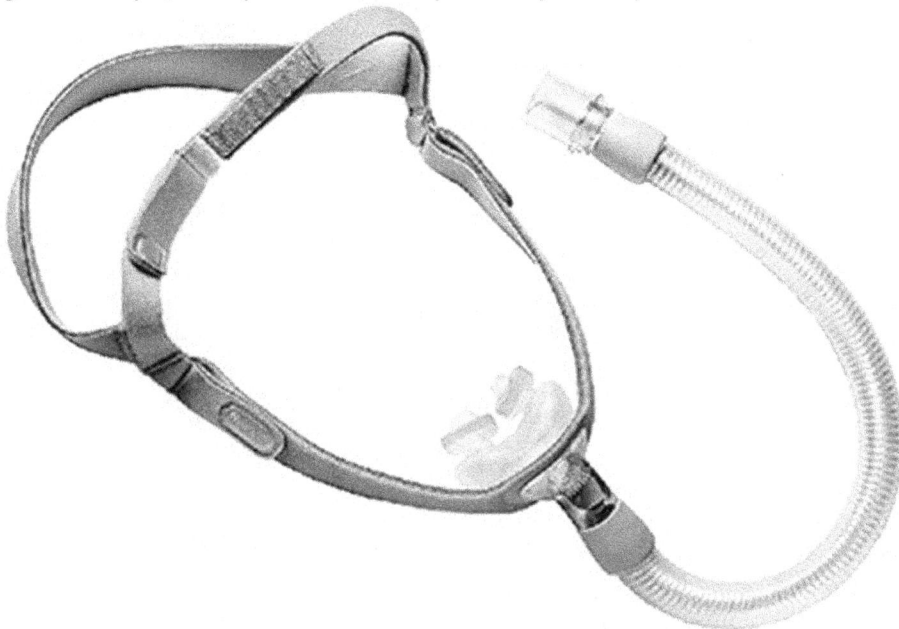

Courtesy of Philips Respironics
Figure 3.5 Philips Respironics Nuance Pro Gel Nasal Pillow Mask.

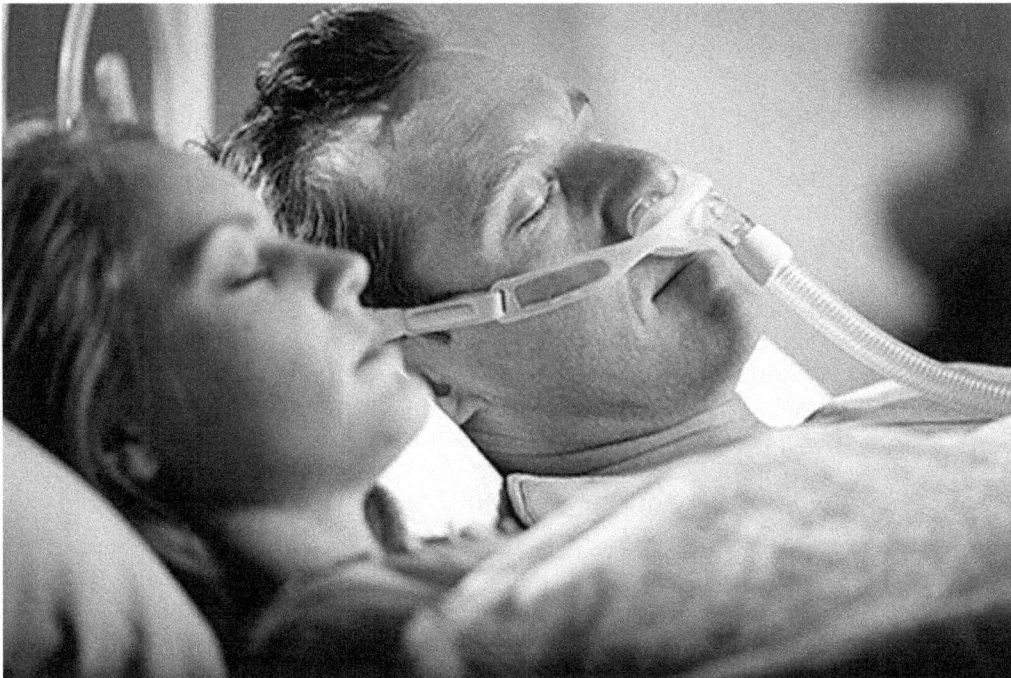

Courtesy of Philips Respironics
Figure 3.6 A sleep apnea patient, wearing Philips Respironics mask along with CPAP Machine.

IMPORTANT TIPS ON NASAL PILLOWS MASKS

(i) You need to tailor your own cloth covers for the mask, wrapping around the straps.

(ii) Or, you can use children's socks as covers so that you can easily cover and uncover the straps by unpeeling the velcros (Each strap can be covered with one children's sock). Please remove the covers from the straps and wash and dry them once every week or every fortnight and cover the straps back. If you develop a habit of doing so, your mask lasts long (for years), and you don't have to purchase CPAP mask once every few months. Expensive sanitizers to clean the CPAP mask and hoses are unnecessary!

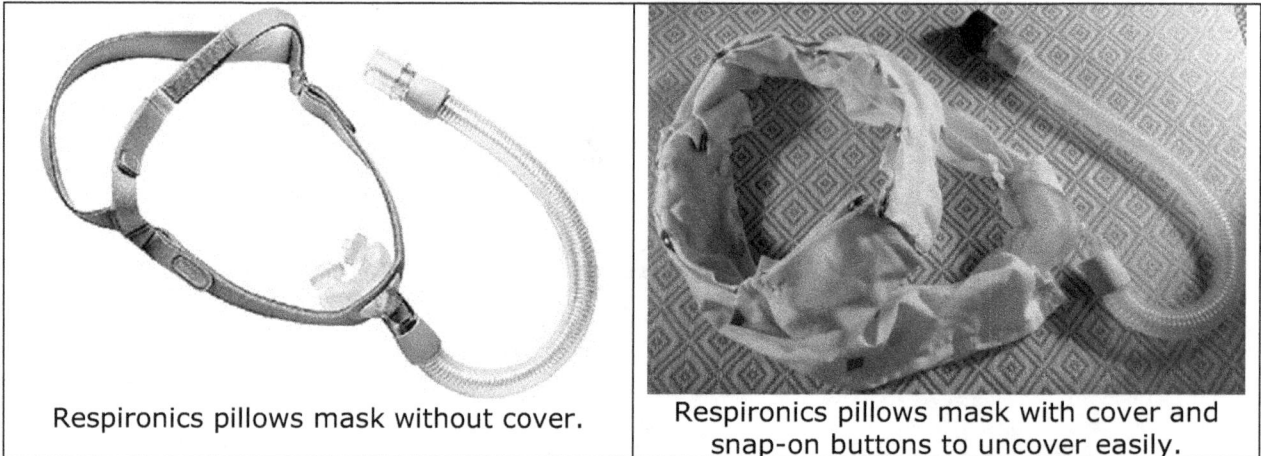

Respironics pillows mask without cover.

Respironics pillows mask with cover and snap-on buttons to uncover easily.

Figure 3.7 A nasal pillows mask would last longer if you tailor a cloth cover around the straps.

(ii) The nasal pillows cushions of the mask seal your nostrils smoothly and comfortably whenever you wear CPAP mask on your face, and are available in three sizes (large, medium & small). It is important that you should wash and clean the pillows cushion every day when you wake up in the morning, at first with warm soapy water, and then with warm water, and then wipe it with a clean towel so that it would be ready for the following night when you sleep with your CPAP machine. You should do that every day. Please do not use antibacterial wipes or disinfecting wipes to clean your nasal pillows cushion (If you do so, you could be swallowing traces of harmful chemicals).

(iii) Every morning when you wake up, you also need to pull out the humidifier from the CPAP machine (while pulling out, press down the right side of the chamber with your thumb), discard the remaining water and wash it with hot water first, and then rinse it with distilled water (or purified water with zero TDS level), and then refill it with distilled water to the maximum level, and then slide it into the CPAP machine so that it would be ready for the following night when you sleep with your CPAP machine. Never refill the humidifier with tap water, as tap water may contain contaminants and dissolved salts, and may enter the air you breathe from the mask.

HOW TO USE A CONNECTOR (SWIVEL ADAPTER)?

STOPPING LEAKS IS OF PARAMOUNT IMPORTANCE IN THE CPAP THERAPY

◉ A sleep apnea patient who is undergoing the CPAP therapy, while using the CPAP machine, must understand thoroughly and practice it with patience on how to connect the heated tube and mask by means of a suitable connector (swivel adapter) to avoid air leaks.

◉ Any air leak would lower the CPAP pressure and would adversely affect on the performance of the CPAP therapy, and may generate wrong sleep report by the end of the night. You cannot simply rely on that sleep report if there are leaks in the air passage.

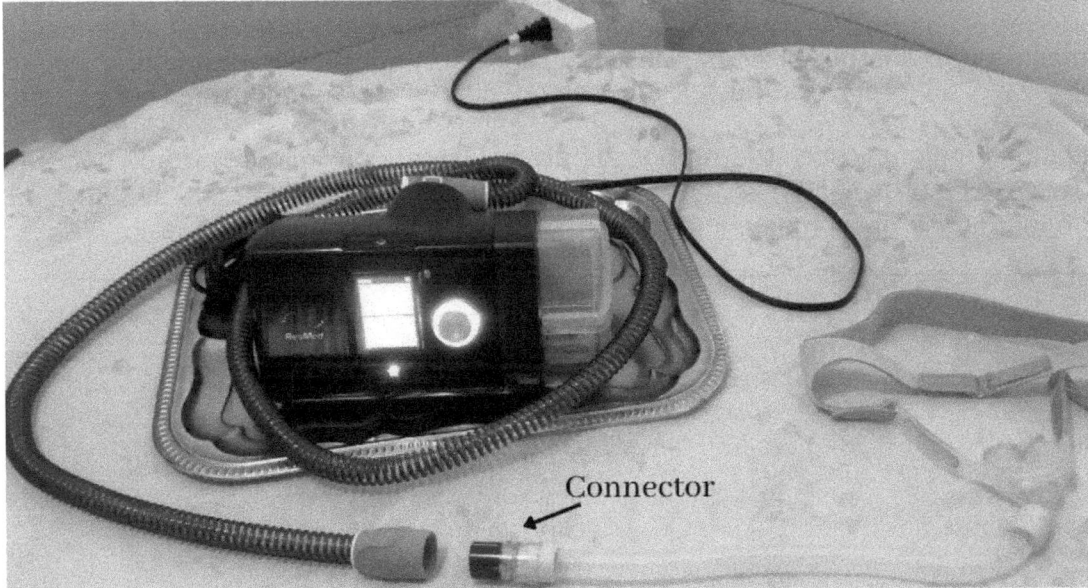

Figure 3.8 The connector (swivel adapter) from the mask is not yet connected to the tube.

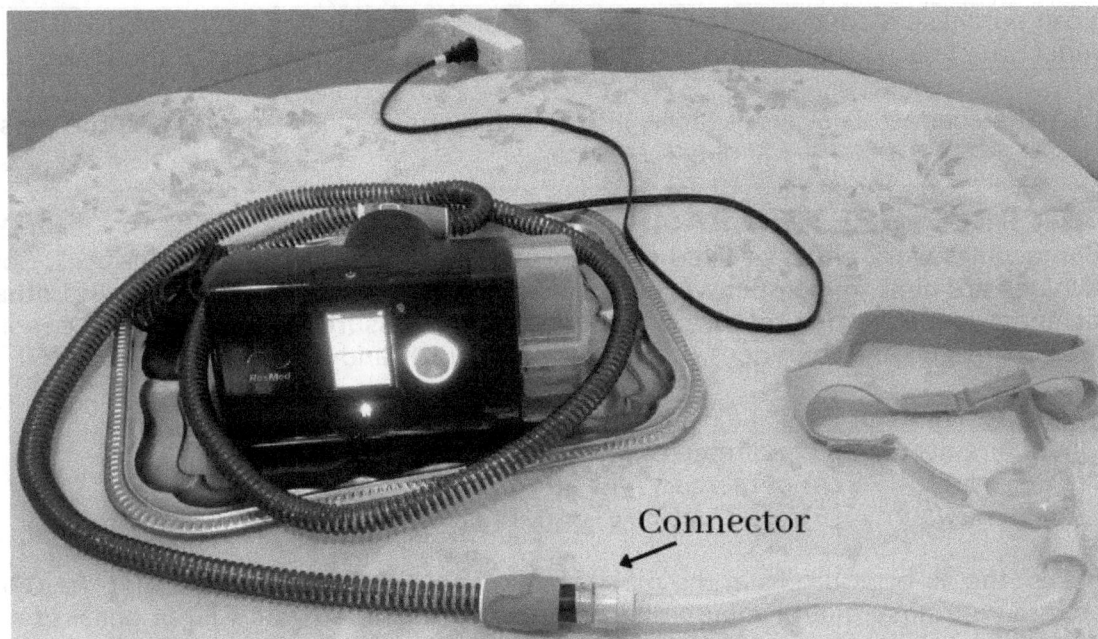

Figure 3.9 The connector (swivel adapter) from the mask is connected to the tube.

REASONS OF AIR LEAKS WHILE USING THE CPAP MACHINE

(i) If there is air leak, check the pillows cushion. The pillows cushion (if you are using nasal mask) was not immersed correctly into the frame, not positioned properly and not sealed perfectly. Also tighten the straps if the mask is not fitting on your face tightly. Check and make sure that there is no opening to escape air.

(ii) Or, the connector (swivel adapter) between the heated tube and mask is probably not sealed perfectly, or even detached. Check the connector, and use an "electrical tape" to tighten the loose connection.

Wrap a piece of "electrical tape" around the edge of the mask tube and push it into the connector (swivel adapter) to ensure a good seal so that air will not leak out while passing into the mask. Wrap another piece of "electrical tape" around the other edge of the connector (swivel adapter), and push it into the opening of the heated tube (hose).

After sleeping overnight, check the rate of the air leak (liters per minute) from your "Sleep Report." By checking the "Sleep Report," you should make sure that air leak is under 24 liters per minute for a nasal mask, and 36 liters per minute for a full face mask. [30, 31]

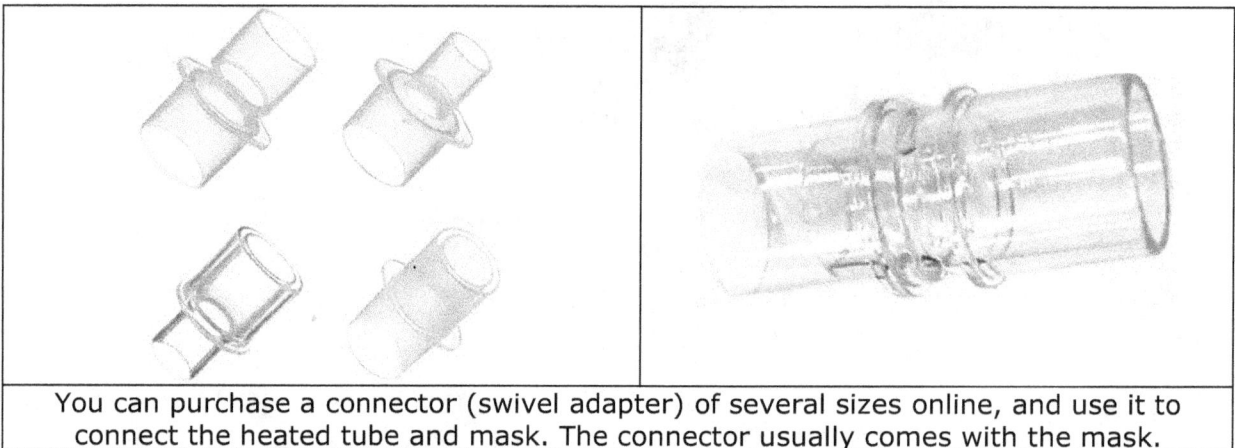

You can purchase a connector (swivel adapter) of several sizes online, and use it to connect the heated tube and mask. The connector usually comes with the mask.

Figure 3.10 The connector (swivel adapter) between the heated tube (hose) and the mask.

+++

CPAP AIR PRESSURE AND RAMP PRESSURE

The CPAP machines work either at fixed pressure or varied pressure (ramp pressure). Some CPAP machines are built to maintain very low fixed air pressure at 6 cm of H2O. And other CPAP machines work at ramp pressure. For example the pressure ramps up from 7 cm of H2O to 11 cm of H2O, and then goes down to 7 cm of H2O, and the cycle repeats.

To understand the units of CPAP's air pressure, here are the conversion factors:
1 atmosphere = 1 atm = 76 cm of mercury = 1033.25 cm of water
1033.25 cm of water = 76 cm of mercury = 1 atmosphere =1 atm
Therefore 6 cm of water = (6)/(1033.25)(76) = 0.44 cm of Mercury = 0.0058 atm

Which means, the air pressure from the mask is very low! Which also means that the CPAP pumps air into your nose and/or mouth at a very low pressure, so you will not get hurt.

+++

HOW TO USE THE RESMED CPAP MACHINES?

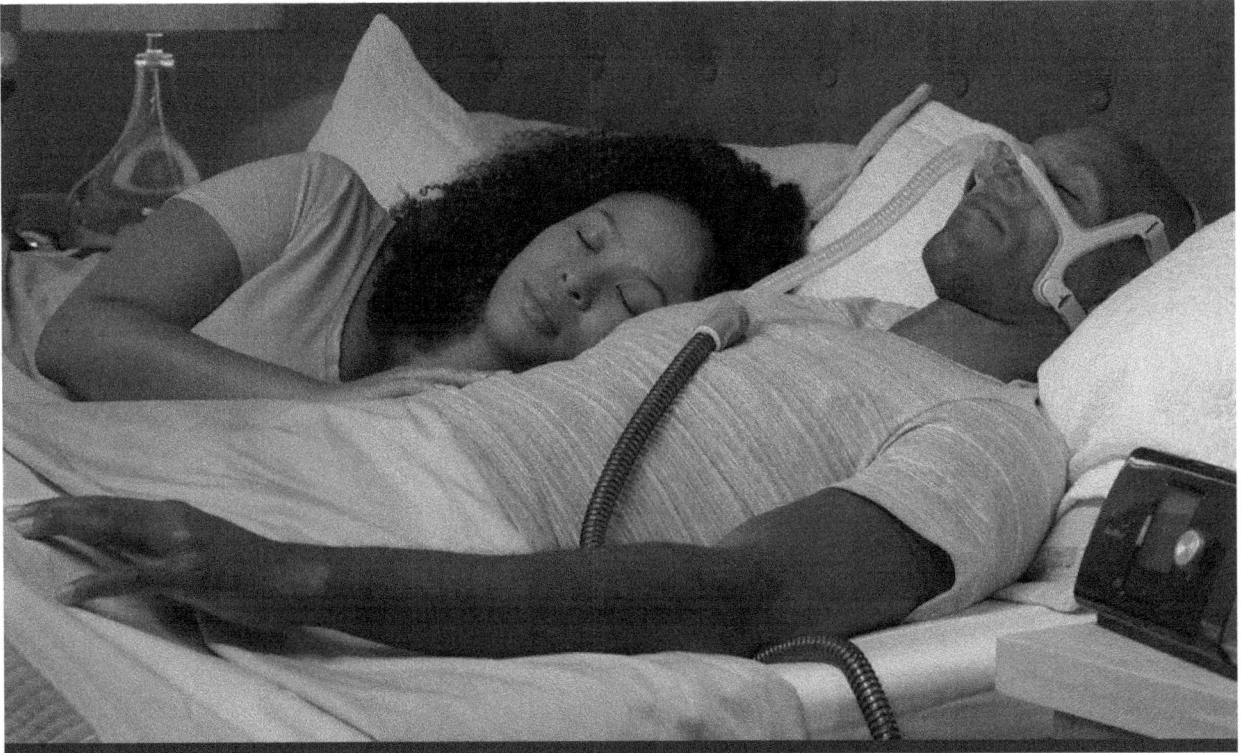

Figure 3.11 A sleep apnea patient is sleeping with the ResMed AirSense 10 CPAP machine.

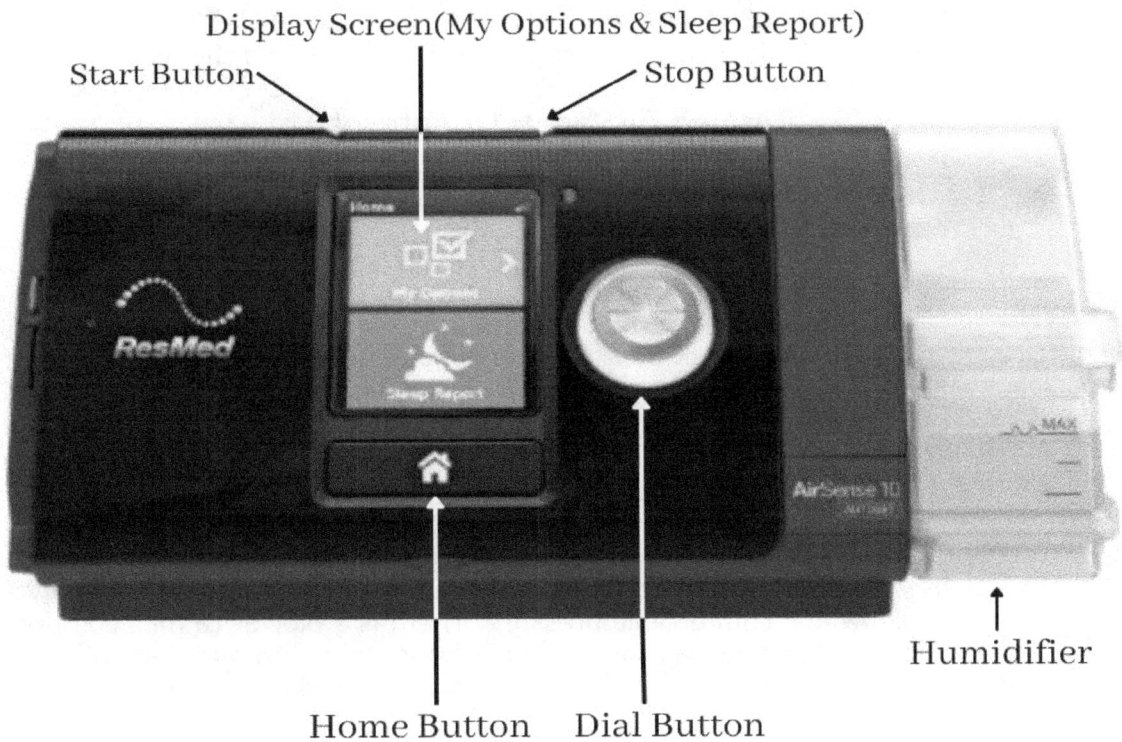

Figure 3.12 The front view of the ResMed AirSense 10 CPAP Machine.

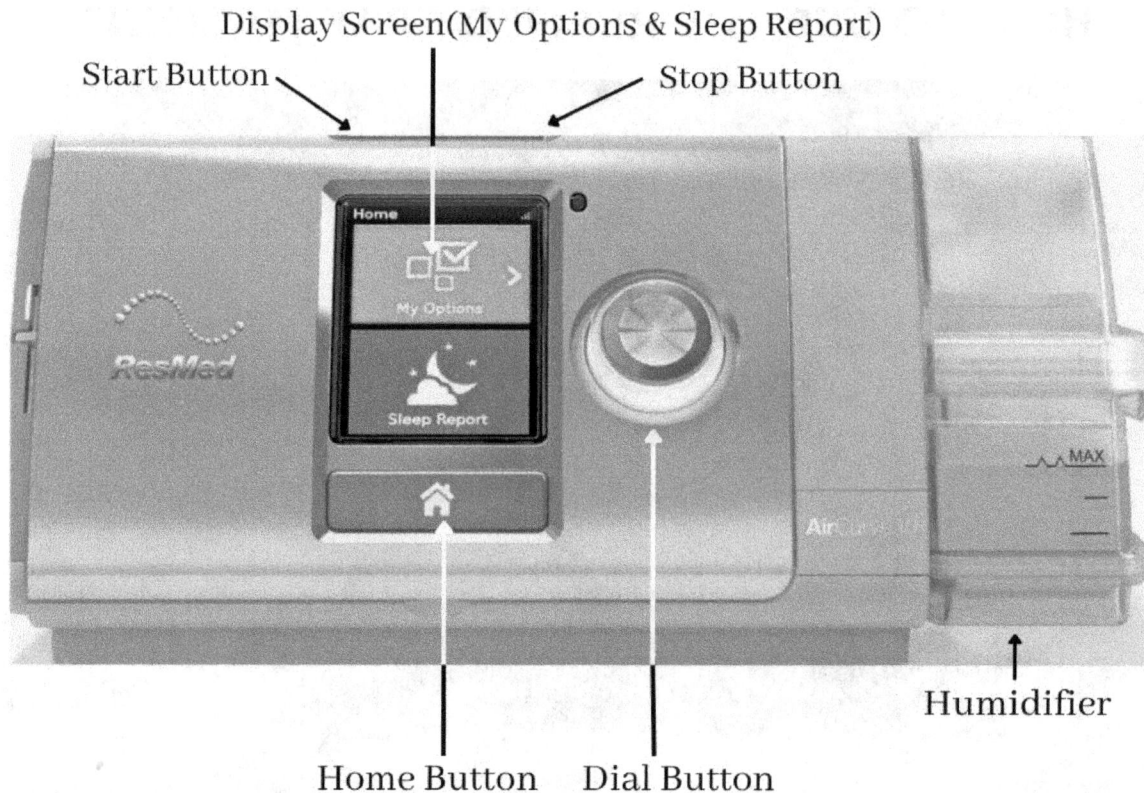

Figure 3.13 The front view of the ResMed AirCurve 10 CPAP Machine.

Front View of the ResMed AirSense 10 CPAP Machine

All the following ResMed CPAP machines have the same front view and the usage instructions are the same:

- ResMed AirSense 10 Autoset
- ResMed AirSense 10 Autoset (For Her)
- ResMed AirSense 10 Elite and
- ResMed AirCurve 10

Dial Button: It is a dial-knob located at the center of the CPAP machine's front view. By turning the dial-button in the clockwise and anti-clockwise directions, you can move from one parameter to another parameter, adjust the value, and control the operation of the CPAP machine.

Home Button with Up-Arrow: It is located on the bottom of the front view. By pressing the Home button or dial-button, you can access the home screen if it is powered off.

Start Button: It is located on the upper-left by pressing which you can start using the CPAP therapy. When you press the start-button, air will be pumped continuously into your throat at a continuous, low and comfortable pressure. There is a blower (a mini compressor) inside the CPAP machine which blows air into your nose and/or mouth and then into your throat during the CPAP therapy throughout the night, depending on what kind of mask you wear.

Front View of the ResMed AirSense 10 CPAP Machine

Stop Button: It is located on the upper-right by pressing which you can stop, interrupt or discontinue using the CPAP therapy anytime during the sleep (usually when you go to bathroom). Whenever you press the stop-button anytime during the night, the CPAP machine stops pumping air and the sleep report shows up automatically, showing you the following sleep report:

(i) Usage Hours
(ii) AHI (Events Per Hour) if it is enabled!
(iii) Mask Seal and
(iv) Humidifier

Whenever you want to go to the bathroom or take a break, you should press the stop-button, then you can remove the mask from your face and place it on your bed, and go to bathroom. After using the bathroom, you can get back to your bed and start using the CPAP machine by simply putting your mask on. As soon as you put your mask on, and whenever your nostrils are perfectly sealed by pillows of the mask, the CPAP machine starts blowing air automatically (if the SmartStart is enabled), and you can see the air pressure being displayed on the home screen. If it is not blowing air automatically, then you can press the start-button to resume the CPAP therapy.

Home Display Screen

● The "Home Display Screen" on the front view of the ResMed AirSense 10 CPAP machine is divided into two parts:

(i) My Options, and
(ii) Sleep Report

● By turning the dial-button in the clockwise or anti-clockwise direction, you can highlight and switch from "My Options" to "Sleep Report," and from "Sleep Report" to "My Options."

My Options [17, 18, 19, 20, 21, 22, 23, 24, 25, 26, 27, 28]

● When you switch to "My Options," and press dial-button, you will see 10 or more parameters to control the CPAP therapy. All 10 parameters are explained below:

(i) Ramp Time	Auto
(ii) Climate Ctrl	Auto
(iii) Tube Temp	27°C
(iv) Humidity Level	4 to 8
(v) SmartStart	On
(vi) Mask Type	Pillows
(vii) Run Mask Fit	>
(viii) Run Warmup	>
(ix) Airplane Mode	Off
(x) About	>

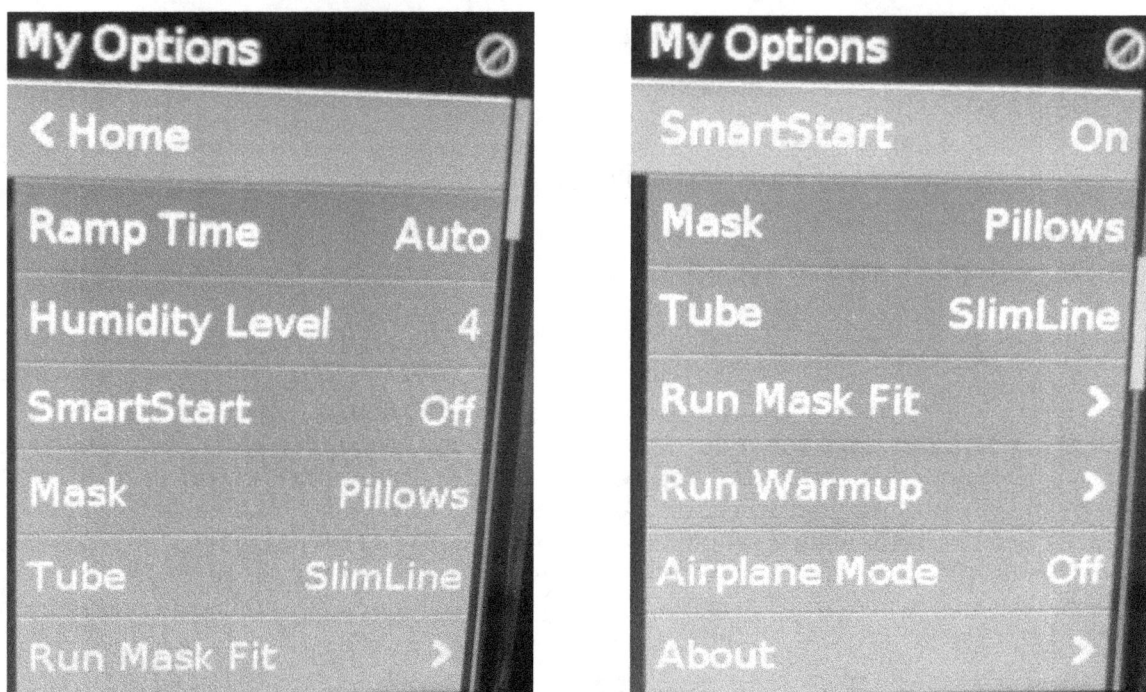

Figure 3.14 The front view of the ResMed AirSense 10 CPAP Machine.

(i) Ramp Time

Ramp time is the period during which the pressure increases (ramps up) from a low start pressure to the prescribed treatment pressure. A patient/therapist can set the ramp time to off, 5 to 45 minutes, or Auto. In order to change the ramp time, you need to go to Setting Menu, and change the ramp time (it is explained below how to do that).

Recommendation: Set this Ramp Time to "Auto."

(ii) Climate Control (Climate Ctrl) [21, 22, 23, 24, 25]

Climate Control is an intelligent system that controls the humidifier and the ClimateLineAir heated air tubing to deliver constant and comfortable temperature and humidity levels during the CPAP therapy. It is highly recommended for all sleep apnea patients that a standard tube should be replaced by a heated tube, as heated tube will prevent condensation and water droplets from getting into your mask. It is designed to prevent the dry mouth, dry nose and dry throat.

Climate Control can be set to Auto, Manual, or Cancel. If you set to "Auto," humidity level cannot be adjusted, the machine will automatically adjusts the humidity level. If you set to "Manual," humidity level can be adjusted from 1 to 8, or it can be turned off. You may not be able to choose "Cancel," if your CPAP is connected to heated tube. If you want to cancel the humidification, then replace the heated tube with standard tube (standard tube is not recommended).

RECOMMENDED SETTINGS

♦ Climate Control = Auto
♦ Tube Temperature = Auto   If you choose climate control as manual, set it to 27 °C.
♦ Humidity Level (Adjust it between 1 & 8 if you choose climate control as manual).

You need to further adjust the humidity level by trial and error while sleeping. If you feel dry mouth during the sleep, then go to Settings menu, and increase the humidity level to 7 or 8 until you reach optimal humidity. If you feel that the air you breathe is too cold, then go to Settings menu and decrease the humidity level to 5, 4, or further down until you reach optimal humidity.

(iii) Tube Temperature [26, 27, 28, 29, 30]

In Climate Control Auto, there is no need to change anything and it takes care of the tube temperature. If you feel that the air in mask is too warm or too cold, you can adjust the tube temperature that suits your comfort. The tube temperature can be adjusted anywhere between 60-86°F, or between 16-30°C, or turn it off completely. To change the tube temperature, you need to go to Setting Menu, and change the ramp time.

RECOMMENDED SETTINGS

♦ Tube Temperature = Auto   If you choose climate control as manual, set it to 27 °C.
♦ Humidity Level (Adjust it between 1 & 8 if you choose climate control as manual).

(iv) Humidity Level [26, 27, 28, 29, 30]

An air conditioner decreases the amount of moisture in the air whereas a humidifier increases the moisture in the air. Household humidifiers are most commonly used to add moisture into the air inside a room. Humidifiers help feel warmer in the winter, kill and destroy air-borne viruses in the room, reduce dry mouth, dry throat and dry skin, reduce nasal stiffness and nasal congestion, and make you feel comfortable and healthy when breathe in and breathe out the air in a room. ResMed introduced this concept into their CPAP machine by adding a humidifier.

The ResMed CPAP machine is equipped with a humidifier which humidifies or moistens the air before delivering it to the mask so that a sleep apnea patient feels cozy while breathing in and breathing out the air. If you feel dry mouth, dry tongue, dry nose, or dry throat, then turn up the humidity level (more moisture will be added to the heated air you breath). On contrary, if you are feeling cold and getting too much moisture into your mask and therefore into your breath, just turn down the humidity level (less moisture will be added to the heated air you breath). You can set the humidity level off, or between 1 and 8 where 1 is the lowest humidity setting and 8 is the highest humidity setting. In order set the humidity level off, you need to use the standard tube (not heated tube). With heated tube, you cannot turn off the humidity. In order to change the humidity level, you need to go to Setting Menu, and change the humidity level (it is explained below how to do that). If you find that the humidifier is not properly humidifying the air, then consider purchasing a new "ClimateLineAir heated air tubing," which delivers the air at controlled temperature and therefore at controlled humidity, and the patient feels comfortable while breathing in.

(v) SmartStart

When SmartStart is enabled, the CPAP therapy starts automatically when you breathe into your mask. When you remove the mask, it stops pumping air automatically after a few seconds. Whenever you want to go to the bathroom, you just remove the mask from your face and pace it on your bed, the air flow will stop automatically (if it doesn't stop, just press stop button). When you get back to the bed after using bathroom, you put your mask on, and the machine starts pumping air automatically (if it does not start, just press start button).

(vi) Mask Type

This option shows what type of CPAP mask you are using. You need to input the type of the mask you are using in Settings menu. If you change your mask to another type, you need to go to Settings menu, and select the appropriate mask name. Then it will show up on the Options menu.

(vii) Run Mask Fit

Mask Fit option is designed to help you access and identify possible air leaks in and around your CPAP mask. To check the Mask Fit, just turn your dial-button to Mask Fit option, and press the dial-button. It will show you the status as Good (green smiley) or Bad (red smiley). If it says good, you don't need to take any action. If it shows red smiley, then you should immediately take action, and fix the mask leak until you stop all leaks. Press dial-button again to get out of this Mask Fit option.

(viii) Run Warmup

Run Warmup option allows you to pre-heat the water before starting the therapy, so that the air is not too cold or too dry at the beginning of the therapy.

(ix) Airplane Mode

Airplane Mode option is used if you are travelling in a plane with your CPCP machine to continue your CPAP therapy. While traveling, before going to airport, empty the humidifier's water tub and keep the humidifier with the CPAP machine (do not detach the humidifier). You must use the CPAP machine with the humidifier in air plane without water in it. Because the CPAP machine is a health device for sleep apnea, it is allowed by most airliners, as it meets the federal government regulations.

(x) EPR (Expiratory Pressure Relief)

EPR™ maintains the optimal therapy for the sleep apnea patient while inhaling and reduces pressure during exhalation. AutoSet offers gentler pressure increases and a smoother night's sleep to help patients with high pressure intolerance. It is usually turned on.

(xi) About

By accessing the About option, you can identify the CPAP machine (the brand name, serial number, model number, SW number, CX number, etc).

Run Hours (Total number of hours spent on this CPAP machine after the purchase):
It is like the odometer for your car. It shows you how many total hours this CPAP machine has been operated till now.

CPAP Life Expectancy: The lifetime of a CPAP machines is approximately 5 years or 15,000 hours. Sometimes you can continue using it even until and beyond 20,000 hours if the machine has no issues.

Sleep Report [17, 18, 19, 20, 21, 22, 23, 24, 25, 26, 27, 28]

● It is very important that a sleep apnea patient must check the sleep report several times during the night (or whenever you wake up from your sleep during the night), and make sure that the CPAP machine is working perfectly. All parameters must make sense while seeing and reading the sleep report. If anything doesn't make sense, the CPAP machine must be taken to the provider or CPAP vendor, and get it recalibrated or fixed.

● When you switch to "Sleep Report," and press dial-button, you will see the following 4 parameters by reading which you can understand the performance of that night's CPAP therapy.

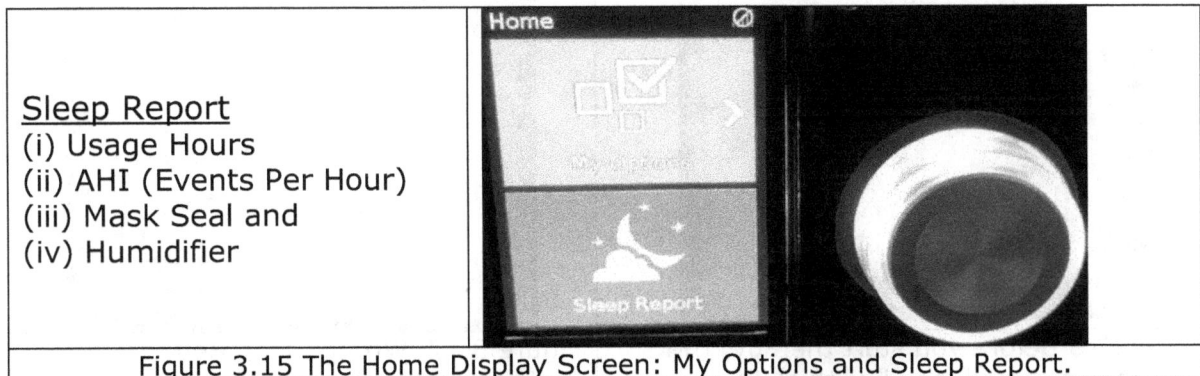

Sleep Report
(i) Usage Hours
(ii) AHI (Events Per Hour)
(iii) Mask Seal and
(iv) Humidifier

Figure 3.15 The Home Display Screen: My Options and Sleep Report.

(i) Usage Hours: "Usage Hours" must be counted only when the mask is "on" to your face or nose. "Usage Hours" is the total time counted only when the mask is sealed to your face or nose <u>from noon of the current day to the noon of the following day (within 24 hours)</u>. By accessing the Settings menu, you should have adjusted the time to your local time. The time in the ResMed CPAP machine must vary from 00:00 to 24:00 hours.

If the mask is "off" of your face or nose for a certain time (for example you spend time in washroom, watching TV, talking on the phone, drinking or eating, staying outside the bed sometimes with the middle-of-the-night insomnia, etc), that time is omitted in the "Usage Hours" being displayed.

(ii) AHI (Events Per Hour): The purpose of CPAP machine is to keep the AHI (Events Per Hour) under 5. Even if you have severe sleep apnea, your CPAP machine must keep AHI (Events Per Hour) under 5. If the AHI is unusually high and showing wrong value, that means the machine needs calibration, you must take your CPAP machine to your provider or CPAP vendor, and get it fixed.

(iii) Mask Seal: If there is "green smiley" next to Mask Seal, that means your mask, tube and connector (swivel adapter) were working perfectly and there was no leak in the air passage during the time you slept. If you see "red smiley" next to mask seal, that means your mask and/or connector had some leak and you must take necessary action to fix the leak or leaks and to make all connections leak-proof. You must learn how to do it yourself without depending on your therapist every day.

(iii) Humidifier: If there is "green smiley" next to Humidifier, that means the CPAP's humidifier is working fine. If you see "red smiley" next Humidifier, that means the Humidifier is not inserted properly or something else is wrong. You need to adjust the settings, or you should get that Humidifier fixed until you see the green smiley.
<u>By checking the "Sleep Report," you should make sure that air leak is under 24 liters per minute for a nasal mask, and 36 liters per minute for a full face mask.</u> [30, 31]

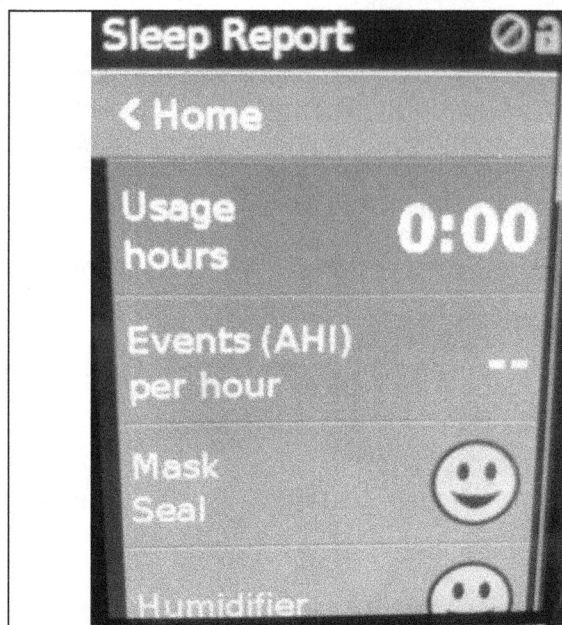

Figure 3.16 Before you start therapy, the sleep report should look like this!	Figure 3.17 Wrong Sleep Report; Something is wrong.

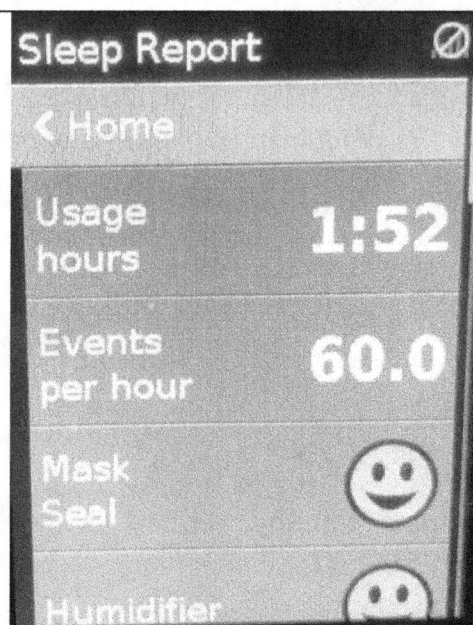

Even though the patient slept for 7 hours, the sleep report showed 1:52 hours, and Events Per Hour is unusually high (60.0), which means the CPAP machine is not working, and something is wrong. Get it calibrated or repaired at the ResMed repair center (Please note that CPAP vendors do not repair CPAP machines).

What Is Clinical Menu or Settings Menu

● You can access, view, and set or adjust various parameters or variables related to a patient's therapy and device configuration by using the Clinical Menu or Settings Menu.

How to Access the Clinical Menu or Settings Menu?

● Therapists everywhere do not allow patients to use Settings Menu, and ask their patients to go to back them if any changes are to be made to the CPAP machine settings, which is not a good practice. Therapists must teach their sleep apnea patients how to use Settings Menu, and how manipulate the parameters in Settings Menu to enjoy good-night sleep.

● HOW TO GO TO SETTINGS MENU OF THE CPAP MACHINE?

Press and hold down both home-button and dial-button at the same time for 3 seconds or until you see "Settings Menu" with an unlock icon on the top right corner of the display screen. If you have successfully performed this operation, you will see that the "Home Display Screen" on the front view of the ResMed AirSense 10 CPAP machine is divided into two parts:

(i) Settings, and
(ii) Sleep Report

And then press the dial-button to see all parameters of the Settings menu.

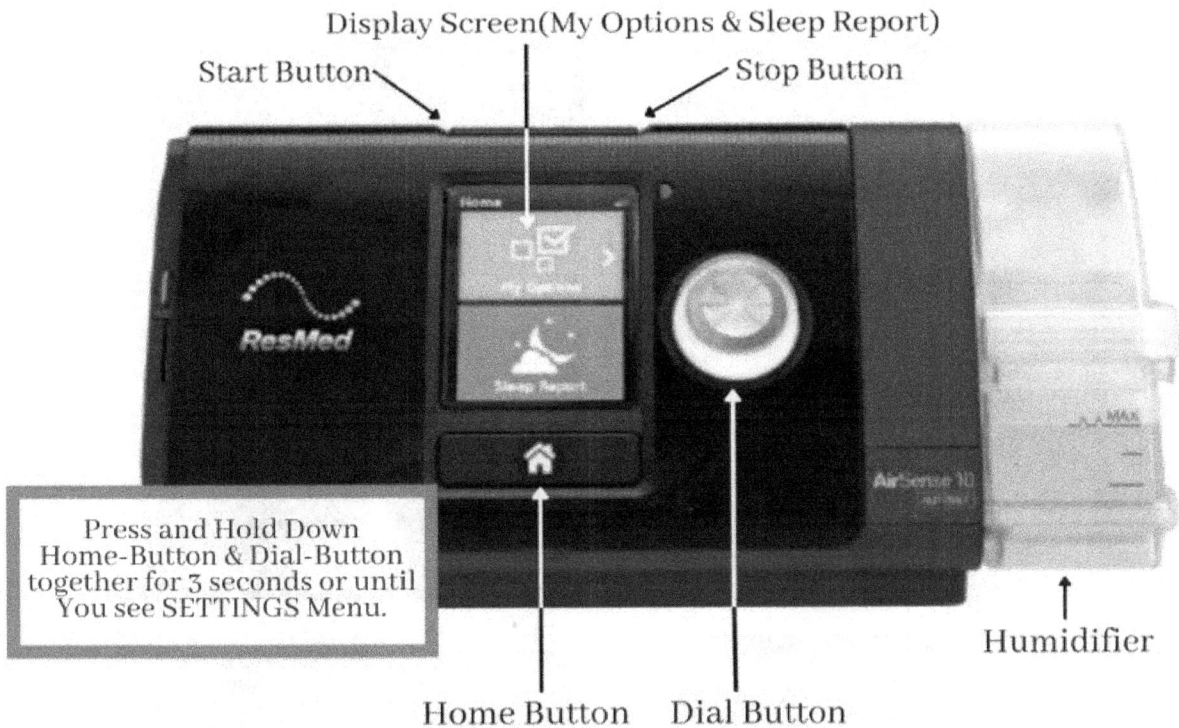

Figure 3.18 How to access the Clinical Menu / Settings Menu?

How to Make Changes in the Clinical Menu or Settings Menu?

● By turning the dial-button in clockwise direction, you can go to any parameter or variable you want on the Clinical Menu, and can make any changes or adjustments that are needed. Some examples are given below on "How to Make Changes in the Clinical Menu."

How to Exit the Clinical Menu / Settings Menu?

● After making changes or adjustments, turn the dial-button in the anti-clockwise direction until your reach blue-colored bar titled "Home." Press the dial-button to reach main screen. Turn the dial-button again in the anti-clockwise direction to reach blue-colored bar titled "Exit Clinical Menu." Press the dial-button again to get back to the original "Home Display Screen."

Table 3.5 Clicical Menu or Settings Menu

Clinical Menu / Settings Menu		Clinical Menu / Settings Menu	
> Home		Options	
Therapy		♦ Essentials	Plus
♦ Mode		♦ SmartStart	On
♦ Max Pressure		♦ Reminders	
♦ Min Pressure		♦ Configuration	
♦ Mask	Pillows	♦ Language	
Comfort		♦ Date	
♦ Ramp Time	Auto	♦ Time	
♦ Start Pressure	4.0	♦ Pressure Units	cmH2O
♦ EPR	Off	♦ Temp Units	°C
♦ Climate Ctrl		♦ Restore Defaults	
♦ Tube Temp		♦ Erase Data	
♦ Accessories		♦ About	

Settings ⊘🔒
< Home
Therapy
Mode — AutoSet
Max Pressure — 11.0
Min Pressure — 7.0
Mask — Pillows
Comfort

Settings ⊘🔒
Comfort
Ramp Time — Auto
Start Pressure — 4.0
EPR — Off
Humidity Level — 4
Accessories
Tube — SlimLine

Settings ⊘🔒
AB Filter — No
Options
Essentials — Plus
SmartStart — On
Reminders — >
Configuration
Language — English

Settings ⊘🔒
Date — 9 Sep 2021
Time — 07:55
Press. Units — cmH2O
Temp. Units — °C
Restore Defaults — >
Erase Data — >
About — >

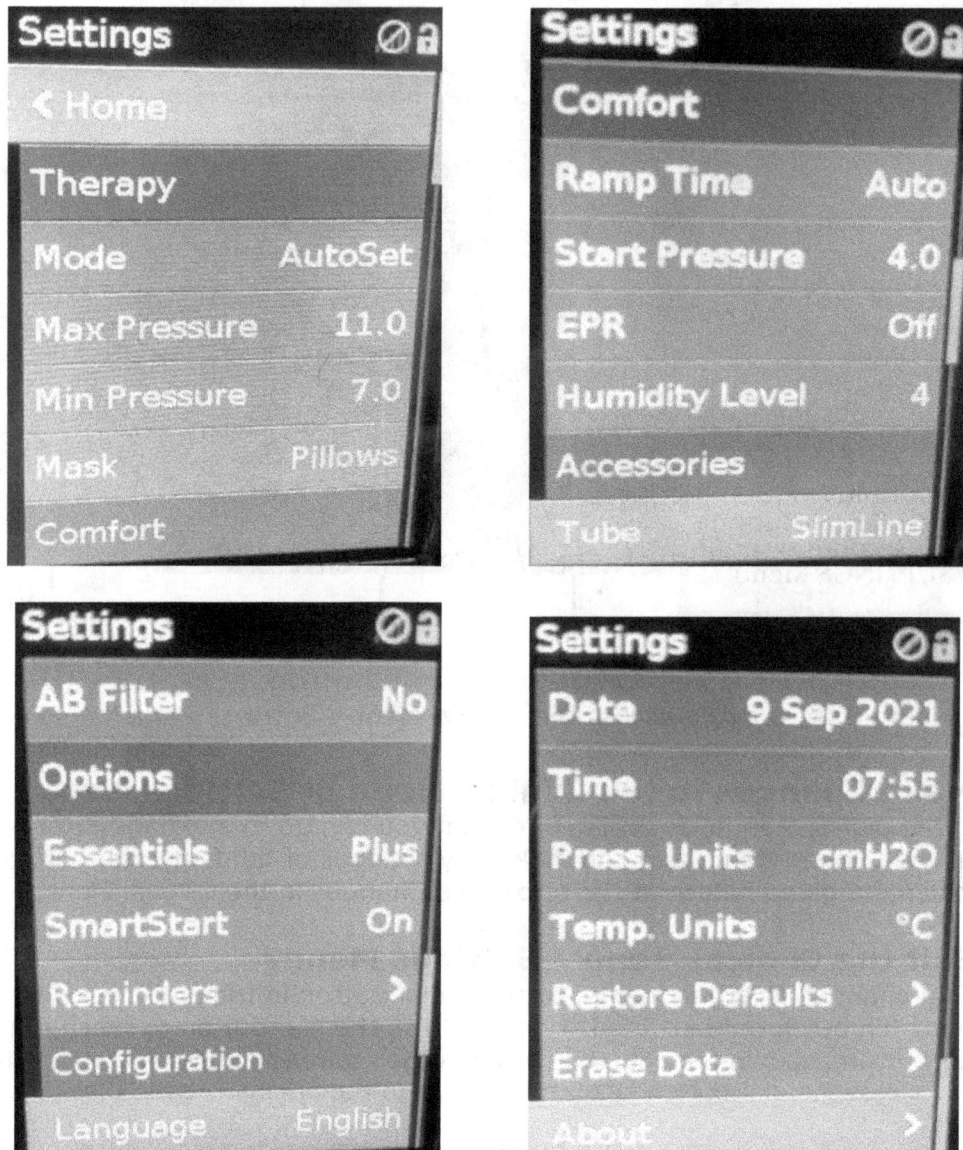

Figure 3.19 Clinical Menu or Settings Menu parameters.

How to Enable and See AHI (Events Per Hour) on the Sleep Report?

• Go to Settings Menu as explained above, and turn the dial-button in the clockwise direction all the way down until you see Date and Time in the Clinical Menu.

• By further turning the dial-button, go to Essentials. Press dial-button when you reach Essentials. There you have two options: Plus and On. You can set to either Plus or On.

• If you set to Plus, you can see AHI (Events Per Hour) in your sleep report.
If you set to On, you will not see AHI (Events Per Hour) in your sleep report.

• After selecting "Plus" in Essentials, turn the dial-button in the anti-clockwise direction, and then exit the Settings menu as explained above.

How to Set the Minimum Pressure and Maximum Pressure?

● Go to Settings Menu as explained above, and turn the dial-button in the clockwise direction down until you see "Max Pressure." Press the home-button. By turning the dial-button, it will allow you to change the pressure to any value you want. Maximum pressure usually is 11 cm H2O. After changing the pressure, press dial-button again to register the desired maximum pressure.

● Turn the dial-button in the clockwise direction to reach the next parameter "Min Pressure." Press the dial-button. By turning the dial-button, it will allow you to change the pressure to any value you want. Minimum pressure usually is 7 cm H2O. After changing the pressure, press dial-button again to register the desired minimum pressure.

● That means the pressure varies from 7 cm H2O to 11 cm H2O during the ramp.

● The starting pressure is always 4 cm H2O.

● After changing the minimum pressure and maximum pressure, turn the dial-button in the anti-clockwise direction all the way to the top until you reach the "Home." And then press the dial-button, you will see the main display screen.

● Turn the dial-button again in the anti-clockwise direction to "Exit Clinical Menu." Then you will be back to the main display screen.

How to Set the Current Date and Time in the Clinical Menu?

● Go to Settings Menu as explained above, and turn the dial-button in the clockwise direction all the way down until you see Date and Time in the Clinical Menu.

● Turn the home-button to "Date." Press the home-button, and set the current date (day, month and year).

● After changing the date, press the dial-button, and turn it to the next item "Time." Press the dial-button, and set the current local time (hours and minutes). <u>You should adjust the time to your local time. The time in the ResMed CPAP machine must vary from 00:00 to 24:00 hours</u>.

● After changing the time, press the dial-button, and turn the dial-button in the anti-clockwise direction all the way to the top until you reach the "Home." And then press the dial-button, you will see the main display screen.

● Turn the dial-button again in the anti-clockwise direction to "Exit Clinical Menu." Then you will be back to the main display screen.

++

How to Erase Data?

● When you try to change the time in Settings Menu, it may not allow you but may give you error message. In that case you need to erase the data before changing time.

● Go to Settings Menu as explained above, and turn the dial-button in the clockwise direction all the way down until you see "Erase Data" on the bottom blue bar. Press dial-button. You have 2 options "yes or no." Select yes, and press dial-button. It will erase data and will give confirmation "Data Erased." Press dial-button.

● Turn the dial-button in the anti-clockwise direction all the way to the top until you see "Home" on the blue bar. Press dial-button again.

● Turn the dial-button in the anti-clockwise direction to "Exit Clinical menu." Press dial-button again. Then you will be back to the main display screen.

● Be Careful: If you erase the data, everything in SD card will be deleted, and your therapist or sleep clinic doctor will not be able to see any of your past activities. You will erase the data only under critical circumstances (if the machine is not working) while adjusting the settings.

++

+++

How to Restore Factory Defaults

● Go to Settings Menu as explained above, and turn the dial-button in the clockwise direction all the way down until you see "Restore Defaults" on the blue bar. Press the dial-button.

● You have 2 options "yes or no." Select yes, and press dial-button. It will restore all default values, and will give you confirmation "Factory Defaults Restored." Press dial-button.

● Turn the dial-button in the anti-clockwise direction all the way to the top until you see "Home" on the blue bar. Press dial-button again.

● Turn the dial-button in the anti-clockwise direction to "Exit Clinical menu." Press dial-button again. Then you will be back to the main display screen.

+++

How to Find Out The Total Usage Hours of Your CPAP

● From the "About," you can see "Total Usage Hours." Press and hold down both dial-button and home-button for 3 seconds or until you see Settings (in place of My Options) on the display screen. And then press dial-button to see Settings menu.

● By turning the dial-button in the clockwise direction, go to the bottom of the Setting-menu until you find "About." Press "About" and read the total number of usage hours.

● Press dial-button to get back to main display screen, and then get back to "Home."

+++

PRECAUTIONS

● Do not plug in your ResMed CPAP machine directly into the power outlet. Always use a surge protector between the power outlet and the CPAP machine.

● Whenever the CPAP machine is not being used, unplug the power cord from the surge protector during the day. Let the CPAP machine is connected the power outlet only during the night when you sleep.

● Every night before using the CPAP machine, make sure that the humidifier is filled with distilled water (do not use tap water) up to the maximum level. Every day when you wake up in the morning, you should dispose the unused distilled water in the humidifier and refill it with new distilled water so that you can use it for the following night.

● Every morning when you wake up, clean your mask with warm soapy water first and then with warm water next. If you use a nasal pillows mask, pillows must be cleaned every day when you wake up in the morning.

+++

OVERNIGHT CPAP PERFORMANCE REPORT IS STORED ON SD CARD

Every CPAP machine comes with an SD Card, already incorporated into the machine, that records and stores all the information about the machine's performance during the night the patient uses it. The custom-made SD Card is capable of recording and storing the summary of the patient's progress every single night. It stores compliance data such as date, AHI (Apnea-Hypopnea Index), CPAP ramp pressure or fixed pressure, total number of usage hours by the patient, mask leak (if the mask is perfectly sealed or if any leaks are identified), mask ON-OFF information (how many times the mask was pulled off the nose) and even the snoring information, in the electronic system called SD Card for up to 365 days. The manufacturer can look back and review the data of a patient's progress throughout the year (if the data were not erased by the user or therapist). By using "Erase Data" instruction from Settings mane, you can delete all the data.

Shown below is the SD Card of the ResMed CPAP machine. As show in the picture, the SD Card is now pulled out. To enable the SD Card function, you just have to insert it into the slot, and close and lock the door to secure the SD Card. The SD Card needs to be replaced at least once every year.

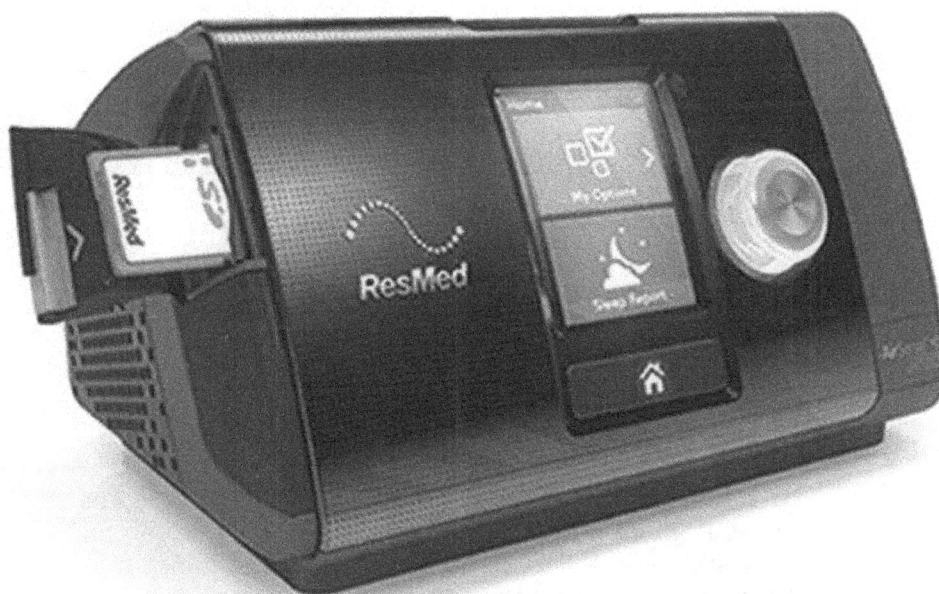

Courtesy of ResMed
Figure 3.20 RedMed CPAP Machine Showing SD Card.

DRAWBACKS OF THE CPAP: (i) The CPAP does not detect and report how many hours the patient has actually slept, and (ii) The CPAP, although it keeps the SpO2 level normal throughout its usage, does not record and display the SpO2 data and chart. If you want to see SpO2 data and chart, you should do the "overnight pulse oximetry test." Even the overnight pulse oximetry does not monitor how many hours the patient has actually slept. Only polysomnogram test monitors how many hours the patient has slept.

RESMED'S MY AIR REPORT

RedMed AirSense CPAP machine users can view their progress report every day a few hours after they wake up. They just have to go to https://myair.resmed.com/ and register to receive the login information (email and password). Every day at around or after 9 am (but before noon), you can access to Myair Report by logging into the website. The online progress report displays the following information for 14 preceding days:

● They allocate 70% of the score for the usage hours (10 points per hour); If you wear the CPAP machine for at least 7 hours, they give you 70%.

● They allocate 20% of the score for mask seal. If the mask is sealed perfectly without any leaks, they give you 20%.

● If the AHI (apnea-hypopnea Index) is under 5, they give you another 5 points.

● If you wear the mask all night long without interruption, they give you 5 points. Every time you go to bathroom, one point is deducted for "Mask (On/Off)." For example if you went to bathroom 2 times during the night, they give you 3 out of 5 points.

They add up all the points you earned, and display it in your progress report. They call it "MY Air Score." You should score at least 90% every day to receive excellent CPAP therapy. If your score is less than 90%, then there is something wrong with your CPAP therapy, and you check your CPAP machine and fix it. If you wear the CPAP for at least 7 hours during the night without a mask leak, your score would be automatically more than 90%. The following is a typical example of Dr. RK when he used his CPAP therapy.

Table 3.6 My Air Score

Task	Score Earned
Usage Hours = 9:32	70/70
Mask Seal: Good?	20/20
AHI = 3 (under 5)	5/5
Mask (ON/OFF)	3/5
Your MyAir Score (TOTAL)	98/100

My Air Score = 98% (Which means EXCELLENT!)

DRAWBACK OF THE RESMED'S MYAIR REPORT:
They give you 70% of the score just for wearing the CPAP. Even if you do not sleep, and even if you suffer from insomnia all night long, they still give you 70% for wearing, which is not a good strategy. They should detect how many hours you slept, and make sure you slept at least 4 hours. If you slept less than 4 hours, they should give you zero, and encourage you to sleep well.

HOW TO KNOW IF THE CPAP MACHINE IS WORKING OR NOT?

● Every morning when you wake up, you should eagerly check your "Sleep Report" being displayed on the ResMed CPAP machine. The most important information you should eagerly look for is AHI (Apnea Hypopnea Index). AHI should be normal (under 5) if the CPAP machine is working perfectly. The purpose of the CPAP therapy is to keep your AHI under 5. If your AHI is normal, that means you had a successful CPAP therapy during the preceding night. If the AHI is normal, your mean SpO2 would automatically be normal.

● The CPAP machine has the ability to kill all excess apneas and hypopneas, and to keep your AHI (Apnea Hypopnea Index) perfectly normal (less than 5 events per hour). If the AHI is 5 or greater than 5, that means something is wrong with your CPAP machine. You should take your CPAP machine to the vendor and get it tested, and fixed, and make sure it works perfectly.

• If AHI is not normal (under 5), you should take action by adjusting the air pressure by trial and error until AHI is normal. If you increase the pressure too much, you could face side effects such as "the general discomfort, nasal congestion, abdominal bloating, mask leaks and associated noise, and feeling of inconvenience due to high air pressure." By maintaining the appropriate air pressure, you can abolish snoring, and achieve normal AHI.

• When you are experimenting with high air pressures, you should ait leek being displayed on the "Sleep Report." Air Leak should be under 24 liters per minute if you use a nasal mask, and 36 liters per minute if you use a full face mask.

• If you are unable to achieve normal AHI (under 5) on your own, that means your CPAP machine is not working, and needs inspection and repair. Take your CPAP machine back to the CPAP vendor or sleep clinic where you got it. They will recalibrate and fix the problem developed.

HOW TO KNOW IF THE CPAP THERAPY IS WORKING OR NOT?
How To Know if Your Sleep Apnea Is Improved or Worsened?
ANSWER: Take the "overnight pulse oximetry test" before and after the therapy, and compare the results (Desaturation Index and mean SpO2).

(i) <u>Take control of your health into your own hands</u>. Do not depend on hospitals, doctors, nurses, or CPAP vendors who can do the "overnight pulse oximetry test" for you. Do your own test, and learn how to do it confidently on your own if you want to reverse or improve your sleep apnea.

(ii) Purchase and learn how to use the Philips Respironics Pulse Oximeter, or Nonin Pulse Oximeter, ResMed Oximeter, Wrist Pulse Oximeter, or any other pulse oximeter to do "overnight pulse oximetry test." Do not rely on cheap devices (they could generate misleading results, so test the device before using it).

(iii) When you get up in the morning after completing the "overnight pulse oximetry test," you should plug in your pulse oximeter to the USB-drive of your computer, upload the data from pulse oximeter to your computer. The computer program generates the report, and displays it on your computer screen. You should focus your attention on two important results when reading the report: Desaturation Index (events/hr), and Mean SpO2 (%). The normal Desaturation Index should be less than 5 events/hr. The normal Mean SpO2 (%) should be more than 95%.

(iv) If the Desaturation Index (events/hr) and Mean SpO2 (%) of the current test are better than the most recent test and all the preceding tests, that means your sleep apnea is improved.

(v) If the Desaturation Index (events/hr) and Mean SpO2 (%) of the current test are worse than those of all the preceding tests, that means your sleep apnea has worsened, indicating that the CPAP Therapy is not working. You should take appropriate steps to improve your results. Either switch to another therapy or lose your excess body weight so that your results and therefore your sleep apnea will be improved.

(vi) <u>If your Desaturation Index (events/hr) is under 5, and also if your Mean SpO2 level and minimum SpO2 are over 95% from the most recent test, that means your sleep apnea is completely reversed</u>.

AHI Versus Oxygen Desaturation Index (ODI)

● Please do not be confused between AHI (Apnea Hypopnea Index) and Desaturation index. AHI (number of sleep apnea events/hr) is used in the daily report of the CPAP machine. You can see the value of AHI every morning on the CPAP sleep report. CPAP machine does not calculate and displays Desaturation Index (number of sleep apnea events/hr). AHI is not the accurate measurement of understanding the sleep apnea progress. Desaturation Index is the accurate measurement of evaluating the sleep apnea progress. Whenever you use the CPAP machine, you should eagerly look for the value of AHI every moring in the CPAP report. Whenever you take the "overnight pulse oximetry test," you should eagerly look for the value of Desatunation Index (number of sleep apnea events/hr) and the value of Mean SpO2 (%).

IMPORTANT NOTE-I

● When taking the "overnight pulse oximetry test," you should not use CPAP therapy (or any other therapy) simultaneously. Please be instructed that, in order to get accurate results, you must discontinue the use of CPAP therapy for at least a week prior to the "overnight pulse oximetry test." Otherwise the use of CPAP therapy influences the true value of your Desturation Index (number of desaturation events per hour), and could generate erroneous or misleading results.

IMPORTANT NOTE-II

● You should always keep in mind that the CPAP does not heal or cure sleep apnea, but only controls it. The CPAP keeps your SpO2 (percentage saturation of oxygen in the blood) level perfectly normal throughout the night as long as you wear it, and as long as the machine is working perfectly without leaks, which is the biggest advantage of the CPAP machine. If you want your obstructive sleep apnea to be improved, cured and/or reversed completely, you need to lose weight until your body resumes normal weight.

How Would You Know If Your Body Weight Is Normal or Not?

● By calculating your body mass index (BMI) or by monitoring your body fat percentage (please refer to Chapter 10 & Chapter 11), you would know if your body weight is normal or not. You should commit yourself to losing weight, and continue to do so until your body resumes normal weight. Even if you lose some excess body weight, you can significantly lower the Desaturation Index (events/hr), and improve your sleep disorder greatly, and feel a lot better. If you could lower your weight to perfectly normal, it is possible to fully reverse the obstructive sleep apnea.

HOW MANY HOURS A NIGHT MUST THE CPAP THERAPY BE USED?

● Research showed that "the average use of CPAP among sleep apnea patients is only 4-5 hours per night, not the recommended 7 1/2 hours a night." [32] Many sleep apnea patients do not tolerate the CPAP machine and noisy mask, and so remove it in the middle of the night, and sleep without it the rest of the night. This kind of habit would lead to adverse and deadly consequences.

● In order to receive the successful therapy, a sleep apnea patient must use the CPAP therapy at least 7 hour a day. To be always on the safe side, if you have moderate or severe sleep apnea, you must not sleep even an hour without CPAP. When a sleep apnea patient sleeps without CPAP, his/her SpO2 level drops to a dangerous level below normal, suffocate himself or herself, and contributes to heart disease, sudden heart attack, and even death.

CHAPTER 3   SLEEP APNEA TREATMENT Section-I
CPAP THERAPY, CPAP MACHINES & CPAP MASKS

REFERENCES

CPAP THERAPY
1. Continuous Positive Airway Pressure, From Wikipedia, the free encyclopedia, Updated and Posted on September 12, 2021.
https://en.wikipedia.org/wiki/Continuous_positive_airway_pressure

2. Colin Sullivan (physician), From Wikipedia, the free encyclopedia.
https://en.wikipedia.org/wiki/Colin_Sullivan_(physician)

3. What is CPAP? by ResMed.
https://www.resmed.com.au/blog/what-is-cpap

4. CPAP Article, Posted by National Heart, Lung and Blood Institute.
http://www.nhlbi.nih.gov/health/health-topics/topics/cpap

5. Spending the First Night Using CPAP Therapy to Treat Sleep Apnea, How to Obtain Your Equipment and Successfully Start Treatment, by Brandon Peters, MD, Medically reviewed by Isaac O. Opole, MD, PhD, Updated and Posted on August 21, 2020.
https://www.verywellhealth.com/spending-the-first-night-using-cpap-3015007

6. APAP vs. CPAP: What Is APAP and How Is It Different Than CPAP?, Written by Daniela Brannon, Updated and Posted on June 14, 2021.
https://www.cpap.com/blog/apap-versus-cpap/

7. What Is a BiPAP Machine and What's It Used For? Medically reviewed by Janet Hilbert, MD, and Written by Carly Vandergriendt, Posted on January 25, 2021.
https://www.healthline.com/health/what-is-a-bipap-machine

8. What is ASV? Treating Complex and Central Sleep Apnea by Kevin Asp, CRT, RPSGT, AAST (The Community for Sleep Care Professionals), Posted on July 27, 2020.
https://www.aastweb.org/blog/what-is-asv

9. What Is ASV? by WeMD.
https://www.webmd.com/sleep-disorders/sleep-apnea/what-is-asv#1

CPAP MACHINES
10. Go to ResMed.com website, and from "Products & Support," select "Full Products Listing," and then you will see: All Products (CPAP machines & Masks) by ResMed.
https://www.resmed.com/en-us/
https://www.resmed.com/en-us/sleep-apnea/
https://www.resmed.com/en-us/healthcare-professional/products-and-support/full-product-listing/

11. APAP vs. CPAP: What Is APAP and How Is It Different Than CPAP?, Written by Daniela Brannon, Updated and Posted on June 14, 2021.
https://www.cpap.com/blog/apap-versus-cpap/

12. Philips Respironics CPAP Machines are available on the following links:
https://www.usa.philips.com/healthcare/solutions/sleep/sleep-therapy
https://www.usa.philips.com/healthcare/product/HCNOCTN447/dreamstation-cpap-bi-level-therapy-systems
https://www.usa.philips.com/c-e/hs/sleep-apnea-therapy/i-currently-use-sleep-apnea-therapy/sleep-apnea-machines

13. Fisher & Paykel CPAP Machines are available on the following link:
https://cpapmachinescanada.ca/pages/search-results-page?q=Fisher+%26+Paykel+CPAP+Machines
Fisher & Paykel CPAP Machines (Listen to Video here)
https://www.fphcare.com/en-ca/homecare/sleep-apnea/cpap-devices/sleepstyle/

14. Fisher & Paykel CPAP Machines on CPAPMachinesCanada.ca
https://cpapmachinescanada.ca/pages/search-results-page?q=Fisher+%26+Paykel+CPAP+Machines

CPAP MASKS
15. Resmed Masks are available on CanadianCPAPsupply.com.
https://canadiancpapsupply.com/collections/resmed-masks-on-sale

16. Philips Respironics Nuance Pro Gel Nasal Pillow Mask, Philips.com
https://www.usa.philips.com/healthcare/product/HC0022500/nuance-gel-pillow-mask

HOW TO USE THE CPAP MACHINE
17. ResMed User Guide for ResMed AirSense (Autoset, Autoset for Her, Elite) CPAP Machine, Print Booklet, 2014.

18. ResMed AirSense Airset and Elite User Manual, ResMed Pty Ltd, 1 Elizabeth Macarthur Drive, Bella Vista, NSW 2153, Australia, June 2020.
https://document.resmed.com/documents/products/machine/AirSense-series/user-guide/AirSense-10-autoset-elite-device-with-humidifier_user-guide_eur1_eng.pdf

19. ResMed Clinical Guide for ResMed AirSense (Autoset, Autoset for Her, Elite) CPAP Machine, 2021.
https://document.resmed.com/documents/products/machine/AirSense-series/user-guide/AirSense-10-device-with-humidifier_user-guide_amer_eng.pdf

20. ResMed Clinical Guide for ResMed AirSense (Autoset, Autoset for Her, Elite) CPAP Machine, 2017.
https://www.resmed.com.au/knowledge-hub/how-can-resmeds-smartstart-setting-help-me-fall-asleep-on-therapy

21. ResMed Clinical Guide for ResMed AirSense (Autoset, Autoset for Her, Elite) CPAP Machine, 2014.
https://www.respshop.com/manuals/ResMed-AirSense-10-for%20her.pdf

22. CPAP Machine Heated Humidifier: Reasons, Indications, and Uses, Written by David Repasky, Last Updated on January 8th, 2021.
https://www.cpap.com/blog/cpap-heated-humidifier-reasons-indications-uses/

23. Why use a humidifier? by ReMed.Com.
http://www.resmed.com/us/en/consumer/airsolutions/air-solutions-support/humidification-faqs.html

24. Signs Your CPAP Machine Is Not Working or Needs Adjusting by Brandon Peters, MD, Medically reviewed by Elizabeth Molina Ortiz, MD, MPH, Posted on May 13, 2020.
https://www.verywellhealth.com/signs-your-cpap-is-not-working-3015051

25. Why Do I Need a Humidifier For My CPAP? by Advanced Sleep Medicine, Inc.
https://www.sleepdr.com/the-sleep-blog/why-do-i-need-a-humidifier-for-my-cpap/

TUBE TEMPERATURE, HEATED HUMIDIFIER AND HUMIDITY LEVEL

26. ResMed User Guide for ResMed ClimateLineAir and ClimateLineAir Oxy(ClimateLineAir is heated air tubing that delivers the desired temperature at your CPAP mack, and ClimateLineAir Oxy is a variant of ClimateLineAir that has a built-in oxygen connector to attach a supplemental oxygen supply), Print Booklet, 2019.

27. ClimateLineAir Heated Tube for AirSense 10 and AirCurve 10 (This Product Does Not Require a Prescription), 1800cpap.com.
https://www.1800cpap.com/climatelineair-heated-cpap-hose-tube-for-resmed-AirSense-10?msclkid=08a2ad7cac601cf79e95cc4dfbc1b30f&utm_source=bing&utm_medium=cpc&utm_campaign=BD%20%7C%20US%20%7C%20Dynamic%20Remarketing&utm_term=2332339040755445&utm_content=Product%20Viewers

28. CPAP Standard/Heating Tubing FAQ's, by Shannon Gibson, Posted on Mar 21, 2019.
https://www.sleepsourcedme.com/post/cpaptubefaqs

29. Humidifier Settings, Support Article Posted by by ResMed.
https://support.resmed.com/en-au/support/humidifier-settings-faqs/

30. A glossary of sleep apnea terms by Sleepvantage.com. The acceptable leak rate is up to 24 litres per minute.
https://www.sleepvantage.com.au/sleep-library/sleep-apnea-glossary#:~:text=Leak%20measures%20the%20amount%20of,to%2024%20litres%20per%20minute.

31. What is considered an acceptable level for CPAP mask leakage (liters/min)?, Air leak should be under 24 L/min if using nasal masks, and under 36 L/min if using full face masks, Quora Discussion Board, October 03, 2019.
https://www.quora.com/What-is-considered-an-acceptable-level-for-CPAP-mask-leakage-liters-min

32. The deadly truth about CPAP: Only using CPAP 4-5 hours a night, considered CPAP success, may prove deadly, Sleep and Health Journal, 2014.
https://www.sleepandhealth.com/the-deadly-truth-about-cpap-only-using-cpap-4-5-hours-a-night-considered-cpap-success-may-prove-deadly/

CHAPTER 4 SLEEP APNEA TREATMENT Section-II

ORAL APPLIANCES AND ANTI-SNORING DEVICES

TABLE OF CONTENTS

CHAPTER 4 SLEEP APNEA TREATMENT Section-II

ORAL APPLIANCES FOR TREATING OBSTRUCTIVE SLEEP APNEA

There are two types of oral appliances:

a. Tongue Retaining Device (TRD)

b. Mandibular Advancement Device (MAD)

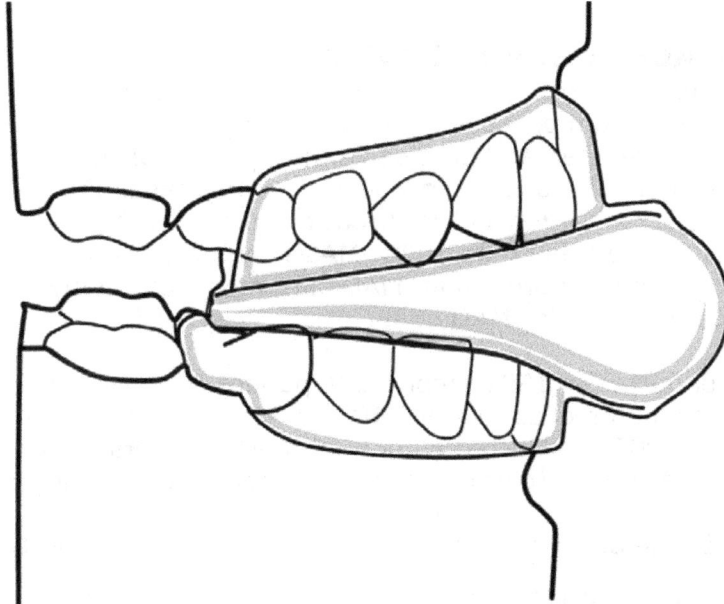

Figure 4.1 Tongue Retaining Device (TRD).

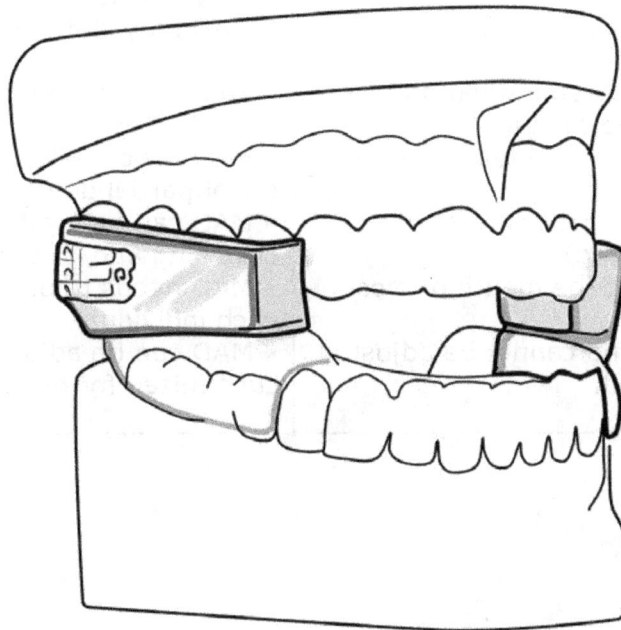

Figure 4.2 Mandibular Advancement Device (MAD).

Tongue Retaining Device (TRD): A tongue retaining device (TRD) in the mouth holds the tongue in a forward position, preventing it from falling backward and blocking the airway. It keeps the airway open so that a person can breathe better, which would help stop snoring. The TRD does not pull your jaw forward or hold it upward, but suctions to your tongue to hold it in place. The device rests between your inner lips and outer gums. You need to breathe through your nose to wear a TRD. For TDRs to work properly, the mouth must be sealed around the oral appliance to sustain the necessary suction. So it is not recommended to open-mouth breathers.

Mandibular Advancement Device (MAD): A Mandibular Advancement Device (MAD) moves the mandible and the associated structure, such as tongue, forward and prevents the tissues from collapsing and blocking the airway. MADs are fabricated so that the lower jaw is more open and protrusive than in the normal biting position. Studies showed that this kind of oral appliance increases the nasal airflow. So there are good chances that the upper airway in the throat could remain open during sleep. Most patients find MADs more comfortable than TRDs. MADs can be custom-manufactured for patients with nasally-compromised breathing. MADs are most commonly preferred devices and there has been a great demand for MADs.

A case study conducted in 1999 among 134 patients revealed that 86% of the patients preferred to use mouthpieces (either TRD or MAD) to control snoring and sleep apnea. Another study in 2005, conducted among 20 heavy snorers, revealed that a low-cost fabricated MAD was a well-tolerated option for both snoring and obstructive sleep apnea.

Table 4.1 The difference between the two oral appliances TRD and MAD. [1]

Tongue Retaining Device (TRD)	Mandibular Advancement Device (MAD)
● TRD pulls your tongue forward.	● MAD works by holding your jaw in a forward position.
● TRD may cause tongue soreness and drooling.	● MAD may shift your jaw and teeth.
● You cannot breathe through mouth unless the device has some holes in it.	● You can breathe through your mouth.
● TRD can be used even with full set of partial dentures.	● MAD is not suitable for people with full set of partial dentures.
● TRD cannot help with bruxism (teeth clenching and/or grinding).	● MAD can help with bruxism (teeth clenching and/or grinding).
● TRD is designed to fit the mouth of most people.	● MAD needs to be custom-designed for each individual.
● TRD design is final and cannot be adjusted after it is manufactured.	● MAD can be adjusted and further customized for maximum efficiency.

LIST OF 41 ORAL APPLIANCES (FDA Cleared)

Table 4.2 The list of 41 oral appliances.

iHATECPAP.Com website claims that the following 41 oral appliances were approved by United States FDA, and can be used to treat mild and moderate obstructive sleep apnea. [2]	
1. Thornton Adjustable Positioner (TAP)	23. Z-Quiet Pro-Plus
2. MicrO2	24. APM Ultra
3. SomnoMed MAS - Dorsal Fin Appliance	25. Hilsen Adjustable Positioning Appliance
4. Respire - Dorsal Fin Appliance	26. Klearway Oral Appliance
5. The SUAD™ Device	27. The Moses Appliance
6. The Temporary SUAD™ Appliance (TSA)	28. OASYS
7. Herbst Telescopic Appliance	29. Silencer System
8. Quali-Som's TheraSom Cast	30. Elastic Mandibular Advancement Appliance (EMA)
9. Tongue Retaining Device (TRD)	31. Medical Dental Sleep Appliance (MDSA)
10. SNOR-X	32. NORAD Appliance
11. aveoTSD	33. Silent Nite
12. Nose Breathe Appliance	34. Snore-Aid
13. Clasp Retained Mandibular Positioner	35. Z-appliance
14. Elastomeric Sleep Appliance	36. TheraSnore Adjustable
15. OSAP	37. CPAP Pro
16. Sleep Apnea Goldilocks Appliance (SAGA)	38. Oral Pressure Appliance (OPAP)
17. Mandibular Inclined Repositioning Splint (MIRS)	39. Sleep Apnea Airway Management System (SAAMS)
18. Nocturnal Airway Patency Appliance (NAPA)	40. SomnoGuard AP®
19. SnoreFree	41. SomnoGuard AP Pro®
20. SnoreGuard	
21. SomnoGuard 2.0	
22. Adjustable PM Positioner	

Table 4.3 The list of best anti-snoring devices

BEST ANTI-SNORING DIVICES Posted by American Sleep Association [3]	BEST ANTI-SNORING DIVICES Posted by American Sleep Foundation [4]
1. SnoreRX Plus	1. SnoreRX Plus
2. Good Morning Snore Solution	2. Good Morning Snore Solution
3. Vital Sleep	3. Sleep Tight Mouthpiece
4. Zquiet	4. Zquiet Mouthguard
5. Sleep Tight	5. Vital Sleep Mouthguard
6. Aveo TSD	6. SnoreMeds Anti-Snoring Mouthpiece

Please do the Google search of the aforementioned oral appliances and anti-snoring devices, read and understand thoroughly, and select the one that suits your mouth and your taste in order to treat your mild or moderate obstructive sleep apnea. Do the "overnight pulse oximetry test" before and after using the oral appliance or device, and compare the results to determine if the appliance or device is working to relieve obstructive sleep apnea or not.

HOW TO KNOW IF THE ORAL APPLIANCE IS WORKING OR NOT?

ANSWER: Take the "overnight pulse oximetry test" before and after the therapy, and compare the results (Desaturation Index and SpO2 level).

(i) <u>Take control of your health into your own hands</u>. Do not depend on hospitals, doctors, therapists, or CPAP vendors who can do the "overnight pulse oximetry test" for you. Do your own test.

(ii) Purchase and learn how to use the Philips Respironics Pulse Oximeter, or Nonin Pulse Oximeter, ResMed Oximeter, Wrist Pulse Oximeter, or any other pulse oximeter to do "overnight pulse oximetry test." Do not rely on cheap devices (they could generate misleading results, so test the device before using it).

(iii) In the first night, you take the "overnight pulse oximetry test" without using any oral appliance or anti-snoring device. When you get up in the morning after completing the "overnight pulse oximetry test," you should plug in your Wrist Pulse Oximeter to the USB drive of your computer, upload the data from your Wrist Pulse Oximeter to your computer. The software generates the report and displays the results on your computer screen. Record Desaturation Index (events/hr) and SpO2 level (%) of this test.

From the value of the Desaturation Index (DI), you can find out the severity of your sleep apnea. For mild sleep apnea, DI = 5 to 14 events/hour. For moderate sleep apnea, DI = 15 to 29 events/hour. For severe sleep apnea, DI > 30 events per hour. Find out if you have mild, moderate or severe sleep apnea. Find out the value of your Desaturation Index (DI).

(iv) In the following night, take the "overnight pulse oximetry test" again by wearing an oral appliance or anti-snoring device. Find out the Desaturation Index (events/hr), and SpO2 level (%). If the oral appliance or anti-snoring device is working, the Desaturation Index should be under 5 events/hr, and the SpO2 level should be normal or at least over 90%.

If your Desaturation Index (events/hr) is more than 5, that means your oral appliance or anti-snoring device is not working. You must find out a better oral appliance or mouthpiece, or switch to CPAP therapy.

HOW TO SELECT AN ORAL APPLIANCE OR MOUTHPIECE?

a. Take the "overnight pulse oximetry test" in the first night without using any oral appliance.
b. Take the "overnight pulse oximetry test" in the following night using the oral appliance (TDR).
c. Take the "overnight pulse oximetry test" in the following night using the oral appliance (MAD).

Then compare the results (Desaturation Index and SpO2 level) in all 3 cases. If the Desaturation Index is under 5 events/hr, that means oral appliance is working. Then compare the results between two oral appliances TDR & MAD, and choose the one that gives lower Desaturation index and higher SpO2 level (%).

REMEMBER: The CPAP machine completely stops a large number of events of apneas and hypopneas, and keeps the Oxygen Desaturation Index (number of events/hr) and SpO2 level (%) perfectly normal. This kind of accuracy would not be possible with oral appliances. You should research and find out if an oral appliance is working for you or not. You may be wasting your time with oral appliance. Your oral appliance probably is not doing anything.

CHAPTER 4 SLEEP APNEA TREATMENT Section-II
ORAL APPLIANCES AND ANTI-SNORING DEVICES

REFERENCES

1. What's The Difference Between MAD And TRD Snoring Aids?, Posted on June 4, 2017, Updated July 2021.
https://www.top10snoringaids.com/whats-the-difference-between-mad-and-trd-snoring-aids/

2. FDA List of Oral Appliances for Sleep Apnea & Snoring, Ihatecpap.com, Accepting New Patients Near Chicago, IL, Nationwide & Worldwide.
https://www.ihatecpap.com/oral-appliances

3. Best Anti-Snoring Mouthguards, Mouthpieces, and Snoring Devices by American Sleep Association.
https://www.sleepassociation.org/top-anti-snoring-mouthpieces-mouth-guards-reviews/

4. Best Anti-Snoring Mouthpieces and Mouthguards of 2021 by Sleep Foundation, Posted on September 14, 2021.
https://www.sleepfoundation.org/best-anti-snoring-mouthpieces-and-mouthguards

CHAPTER 5 SLEEP APNEA TREATMENT Section-III

NASAL STRIPS THERAPY TO IMPROVE BREATHING AND TO RELIEVE MILD SLEEP APNEA

TABLE OF CONTENTS

CHAPTER 5 SLEEP APNEA TREATMENT Section-III

NASAL STRIPS THERAPY TO IMPROVE BREATHING AND TO RELIEVE MILD SLEEP APNEA

There are Two Types of Nasal Strips:
- a. Breathe Right Strips
- b. Sleep Right Strips

NASAL STRIPS HELP IMPROVE BREATHING: If you suffer from nasal congestion and/or deviated septum in which the nasal passages are unevenly displaced (one passage is bigger with swollen nasal tissues and the other passage is smaller), it is very likely that not enough air passes through your nose into your lungs. As a result your blood oxygen levels may fall below normal. In that case, if you use nasal strips, they could instantly open your nose up to 38% (38% wider nostrils could breathe in 38% more air). Nasal strips, by allowing more air to pass through your throat, could help prevent the obstruction in the nose. When the nose has no obstruction, more air would pass through the airway of your throat and your blood oxygen levels (SpO2) would be normal. Although nasal strips are most commonly used to breathe well and sleep well, and to prevent snoring. They could also help treat mild obstructive sleep apnea because they could keep your nose fully open, and you can inhale more air.

Watch YouTube Demontrations On How to Use Nasal Strips [3, 4]
https://www.youtube.com/watch?v=t1pW6gVXDUY
https://www.youtube.com/watch?v=K67ycbo8giw

BREATHE RIGHT STRIPS [1]

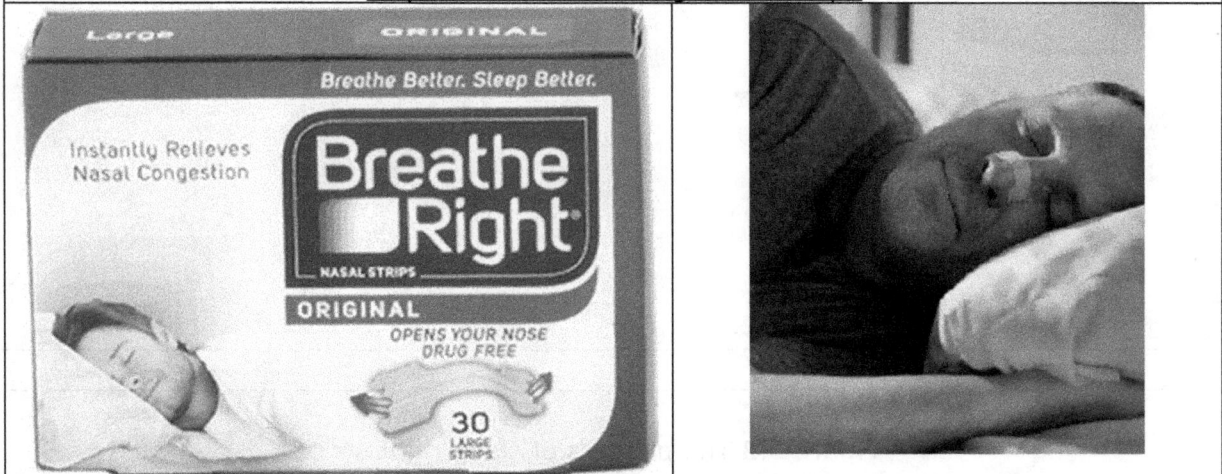

Courtesy of Breatheright.com
Figure 5.1 The pictures of breathe right strips.

SLEEP RIGHT STRIPS [2]

Please visit the following website to learn all about sleep right strips:
http://www.sleepright.com/nasal-breathe-aid/

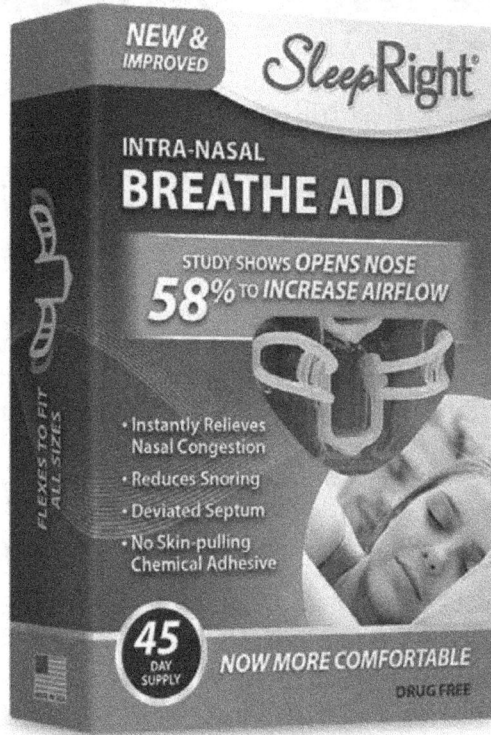

Courtesy of SleepRight.Com

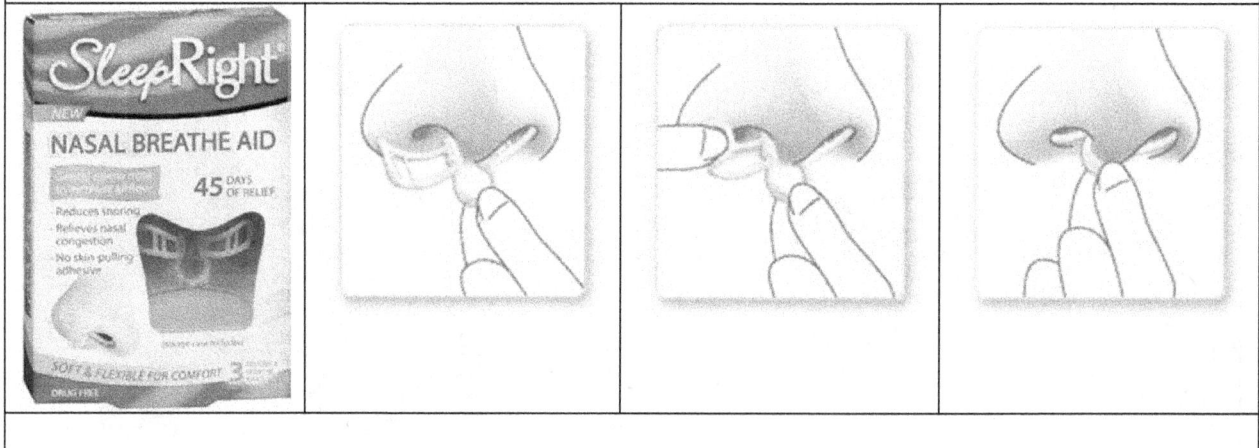

Figure 5.2 The pictures of sleep right strips.

HOW TO KNOW IF THIS TREATMENT IS WORKING OR NOT?

ANSWER: Take the "overnight pulse oximetry test" before and after the therapy, and compare the results (Desaturation Index and mean SpO2).

(i) <u>Take control of your health into your own hands</u>. Do not depend on hospitals, doctors, nurses, or CPAP vendors who can do the "overnight pulse oximetry test" for you. Do your own test, and learn how to do it confidently on your own if you want to reverse or improve your sleep apnea.

(ii) Purchase and learn how to use the Philips Respironics Pulse Oximeter, or Nonin Pulse Oximeter, ResMed Oximeter, Wrist Pulse Oximeter, or any other pulse oximeter to do "overnight pulse oximetry test." Do not rely on cheap devices (they could generate misleading results, so test the device before using it).

(iii) When you get up in the morning after completing the "overnight pulse oximetry test," you should plug in your pulse oximeter to the USB-drive of your computer, upload the data from pulse oximeter to your computer. The computer program generates the report, and displays it on your computer screen. You should focus your attention on two important results when reading the report: (i) Desaturation Index (events/hr), and (ii) Mean SpO2 (%).The normal Desaturation Index should be less than 5 events/hr. The normal Mean SpO2 (%) should be more than 95%.

(iv) If the Desaturation Index (events/hr) and Mean SpO2 (%) of the current test are better than the most recent test and all the preceding tests, that means your sleep apnea is improved. If these results are worse than those of all the preceding tests, that means your sleep apnea has worsened. You should take appropriate steps (switch to another therapy or lose your excess body weight) to improve your results (i) Desaturation Index (events/hr), and (ii) Mean SpO2 (%).

(v) If your Desaturation Index (events/hr) is under 5, and also if your Mean SpO2 level is over 95% <u>from an "overnight pulse oximetry test," without using any nasal strip</u>, that means your sleep apnea is completely reversed. You can accomplish that by losing weight.

If You Don't Have Sleep Apnea

Just try these nasal strips and if you breathe well and sleep well while wearing these strips, then continue using them.

If You Have Mild Sleep Apnea, How to Select the Right Nasal Strips?

There is no guarantee that the nasal strips would work as good as the CPAP machine to combat and destroy apneas and hypopneas throughout the night while you sleep. That is why you should take the "overnight pulse oximetry test" several times and compare the results to find out which nasal strips are working, and which nasal strips are not working.

HOW TO SELECT WHICH BREATHING STRIPS SUIT YOU?

(i) Take the "overnight pulse oximetry test" on the first night just before you started using the nasal strips. Find out the results such as Desaturation Index (events/hr) and Mean SpO2 (%) in the next morning. Record these values carefully.

(ii) Take the "overnight pulse oximetry test" again on the following night by wearing the Breathe Right strips. Find out results such as the Desaturation Index (events/hr) and Mean SpO2 the very next morning. Record these values carefully.

(iii) Take the "overnight pulse oximetry test" again on the following night by wearing the Sleep Right Strips. Find out results such the Desaturation Index (events/hr) and Mean SpO2 (%) the very next morning. Record these values carefully.

Then compare the results of the three aforementioned tests. If the Breathe Right Strips reduced the Desaturation Index (events/hr) significantly and increased the Mean SpO2 (%), that means they are working and it would be worth purchasing them and using them every night. Also compare the results between using the Breath Right Strips and Sleep Right Strips, and choose the strips that reduced the desaturation events the most, and increased the Mean SpO2 (%) level the most, and stick to those strips.

CAUTION: If you are lucky, these kind of nasal strips help relieve "mild sleep apnea." If you have moderate sleep apnea or severe sleep apnea, these kind of nasal strips won't work. You need much stronger therapy such as the CPAP therapy or oral appliance to relieve sleep apnea. However please do not rely on blind faith without scientific evidence that breath right or sleep right strips would work for you. Take the "overnight pulse oximetry test," and find out if nasal strips are working for you are not. You can very easily find out from the test results.

REMEMBER: The CPAP machine completely stops a large number of events of apneas and hypopneas, and keeps the AHI (Apnea Hypopnea Index) and Mean SpO2 (%) perfectly normal throughout the night when you sleep as long as there are no leaks in your CPAP mask. The CPAP machine keeps your AHI (Apnea Hypopnea Index) perfectly normal means it keeps your Desaturation Index (Number of sleep apnea events per hour) normal as well during the night you slept with the CPAP machine. This kind of accuracy would certainly not be possible with nasal strips. You should research and find out if nasal strips are working for you or not!

An "overnight pulse oximetry test" would clearly reveal if you have mild, moderate or severe sleep apnea. Refer to Table 2.7 in Chapter 2 (shown below for your comfort).

Table 2.7 Assessment guidelines of sleep apnea using desaturation index.

SpO2 Level (%)	Desaturation Index (Events/hr)	Assessment
96% - 99%	0 - 4	Normal
90% - 95%	5 - 14	Mild Sleep Apnea
80% - 90%	15 - 29	Moderate Sleep Apnea
< 80%	≥ 30	Severe Sleep Apnea

CHAPTER 5   NASAL STRIPS

REFERENCES

1. Breathe Right Strips Websites.
https://www.breatheright.com/
http://www.breatheright.ca/
https://www.breatheright.com/faqs/

2. Sleep Right Strips Website.
http://www.sleepright.com/nasal-breathe-aid/

3. Youtube Demonstration on How to Use Nasal Strips (Breathe Right & Sleep Right).
https://www.youtube.com/watch?v=t1pW6gVXDUY

4. Youtube Demonstration on How to Use Breathe Right Nasal Strips.
https://www.youtube.com/watch?v=K67ycbo8giw

CHAPTER 6 SLEEP APNEA TREATMENT Section-IV

NASAL SPRAYS TO IMPROVE BREATHING

TABLE OF CONTENTS

CHAPTER 6 SLEEP APNEA TREATMENT Section-IV
NASAL SPRAYS TO IMPROVE BREATHING

NASAL CONGESTION AND SINUS INFECTION

Nasal congestion or stuffy nose is considered as a symptom of sinus infection. The sinus is a cavity within a bone or other tissue in the bones of the face or skull, connecting the nasal cavities. Nasal congestion and sinus pressure are most probably caused by common cold and/or flu. When you are attacked by cold or flu, your nasal passages become inflamed and irritated and begin producing extra mucus with swollen nasal tissue. In order to thin out the extra mucus, you need to drink lots of fluids or water. Drinking lots of liquids could also prevent the sinus cavities from getting blocked. However drinking lots of fluids may not effectively and quickly treat nasal congestion.

GENERAL TREATMENT USING NASAL SPRAYS

Nasal sprays are used by general public to treat cold, flu and cough. To treat chronic nasal congestion, both the prescription drugs and non-prescription products are available. Three are three types of nasal sprays available as the otc (over the counter) products such as decongestants, salt-water solutions and steroid nasal sprays. [1] Decongestants act against the stuffiness in and around the lining of your nose, and the would be able to breathe better. The salt-water solution loosens the mucus, and the person becomes relieved from clod, flu and cough. When the nose is stiffed up by sinus infection, a steroid nasal spray would quickly relive the symptoms.

How to Use Nasal Spray: Close one nostril by pressing it with a finger, put the tip of the nasal spry bottle into the other nostril that is open, and squeeze the nasal spray into the other nostril so that the limited amount of nasal spray would enter into your nose; Do the same by switching to the other side of the nose. After applying the nasal spray medication into the nose, wait for some time, and do not blow your nose right away and do not sneeze. This kind of precaution would allow the medication to stay inside the nose for awhile so that the healing process takes place, and the relief from nasal congestion can be achieved. The American Academy of Family Physicians [2] recommends that you should blow your nose before using your spray, and do not blow afterwards. Make sure to shake the nasal spray bottle before using it, and to also squirt it into the air a few times, until a fine mist comes out. Always check your nasal spray unit to ensure it hasn't expired.

The most common treatment for nasal congestion and sinus pressure is to use a saline spray, which keeps nasal passages moist and clean. If you have tumors or polyps in your nasal passages or sinuses that are keeping mucus from draining out, you may need to undergo a surgical procedure to remove the tumor.

Nasal sprays may contain one or more of the following ingredients: nasal steroids such as mometasone or fluticasone, antibiotics, decongestants, antihistamines or other ingredients. Nasal sprays help cleanse the nostrils and remove the obstructions in your nose. You would then be able to breathe well and sleep well throughout the night. A clean nose without obstructions also helps keep the airway open in your throat by allowing more air to pass freely into your lungs when you inhale. Which obviously means your Mean SpO2 level (mean value of the percentage saturation of oxygen in the blood) could be improved.

(i) NETI POT [3]

Neti Pot is the simplest device available in the market to treat sinuses and nasal congestion at home. Whether it is a one-time sinus infection or chronic sinusitis, a Neti Pot with a saline solution can help thin out mucus and promote healing. Saline solution is used to treat dry or irritated nasal passages caused by colds, allergies, low humidity and even to treat the overuse of decongestant nasal sprays. Saline spray is a salt solution. It works by rinsing and moisturizing the nostrils. As shown in the picture below, when you go to bed every night, just prop your head up, and pour the saline solution into your nostrils so that your nose is entirely rinsed and cleaned by removing the obstructions. During the time you cleanse your nose, you should not breathe in or breathe out. This nasal spray helps you breathe well and sleep well.

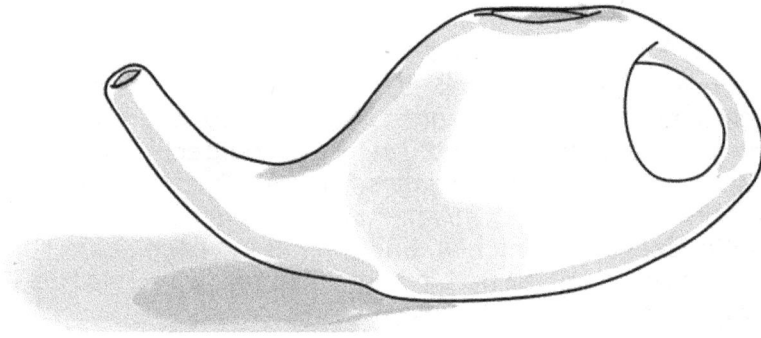

Figure 6.1 The picture of a typical neti pot, most commonly used by people.

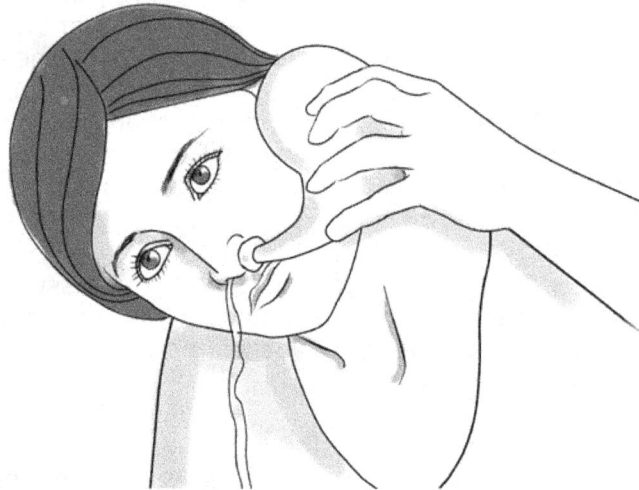

Figure 6.2 A lady is using the neti pot to get rid of nasal congestion.

(ii) Flonase Nasal Spray [4]

https://www.flonase.com/
https://www.flonase.com/products/
http://www.flonase.ca/

Flonase is now available without a prescription over-the-counter (OTC). Flonase Nasal Spray is used to relieve nasal congestion, sneezing, runny nose, itchy nose and watery eyes caused by seasonal or year-round allergies. Flonase Nasal Spray contains fluticasone. Fluticasone is corticosteroid that prevents the release of substances in the body that cause inflammation. Flonase Nasal Spray is being used by adults and children who are at least 4 years old.

Flonase helps decrease inflammation in the nasal tissues, reducing bodily chemicals known as cytokines, which can cause inflammation when a person is exposed to allergens. With Flonase Nasal Spray treatment, you can breathe easy, and get better sleep as more oxygen would enter into your lungs and then into your bloodstream.

Flonase Has Been Used to Treat Obstructive Sleep Apnea in Children [5]

It is believed by some people that the Flonase Nasal Spray could help reduce snoring and can be used as a possible treatment for mild sleep apnea in children. The treatment for sleep apnea in children is very different from that in adults. Children, almost all, cannot tolerate the CPAP therapy. It was reported by some clinical study that the daily use of Flonase for six weeks or longer would cut down the number of oxygen desaturation events per hour, indicating that the sleep apnea symptoms can significantly be reduced with Flonase Nasal Spray treatment. Many of these children have enlarged tonsils or adenoids, and Flonase has helped eliminate the need for a sleep apnea surgery in some children. It was also interpreted that the daily use of Flonase Nasal Spray increased the airway opening of the throat, allowing more air to pass through while breathing during sleep. When more air passes through the airway, the Mean SpO2 level (the percentage saturation of oxygen in the blood) improves, thereby reducing the sleep apnea events per hour. Sleep apnea is a disorder in which the sleeper either breathes shallowly and infrequently, including snoring, and/or has unusually long pauses in breathing.

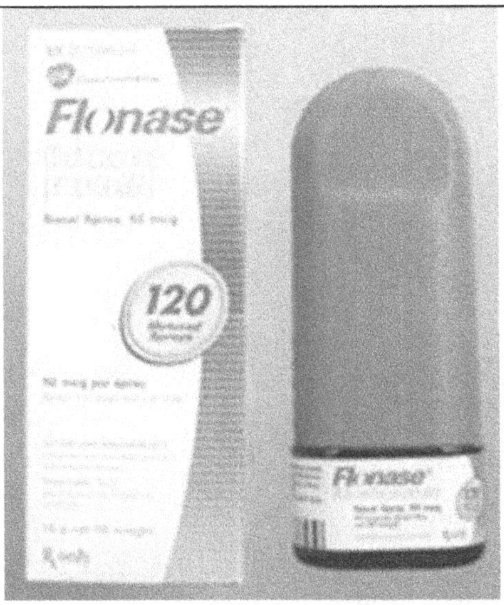

Courtesy of Flonase
Figure 6.3 Flonase nasal spray unit.

Obstructive Sleep Apnea In Children and Adolescents

Obstructive Sleep Apnea in babies, children and adolescents is actually different than the sleep apnea we find and experience in adults. While adults usually have tiredness and daytime sleepiness, children are more likely to have behavioral problems, noisy breathing and snoring. The underlying cause in adults is often obesity. Adults mostly use the CPAP therapy.

Treatment of allergies and sinus inflammation: Medications, such as a steroid nasal spray, saline nasal rinses, and/or other allergy medications, may be an option for children with mild sleep apnea symptoms. These OTC medications can reduce airway constriction and poor tongue posture caused by constantly breathing through the mouth. Allergy treatment could help relieve obstructive mild sleep apnea in children.

ANTI-INFLAMMATORY THERAPY FOR OBSTRUCTIVE SLEEP APNEA IN CHILDREN, CLINICAL STUDY [6]

Anti-inflammatory treatment of childhood Obstructive Sleep Apnea (OSA) is a promising approach that might replace surgical treatment in children with mild OSA in the future or be used as postsurgical therapy for residual OSA. Although a few studies indicate that intranasal corticosteroids and oral leukotriene receptor antagonists have beneficial effects, more information is needed on dosing, duration and long-term effects of these treatments.

(iii) NAVAGE NOSE CLEANSER [7]
https://www.navage.com/
https://www.navage.ca/en/
https://www.navage.com/category-s/53.htm   (Customer Reviews)

The Navage.com website claims that: Naväge is the world's only saline nasal irrigator with powered suction that was clinically proven to relieve sinus congestion due to allergies, sinusitis, hay fever, cold and flu, dry air, environmental pollutants, etc. It works naturally, safely and effectively without drugs but with gentle powered suction. It is powered by 2 AA batteries (included in the package).

Nasal irrigation is a simple, inexpensive treatment that relieves the symptoms of a variety of sinus conditions, reduces the use of medical resources, and could help minimize antibiotic resistance. Nasal irrigation is clinically proven to relieve sinus congestion safely and effectively without drugs. Naväge sets the new standard for personal nasal care with its exceptional convenience, consistency and ease of use.

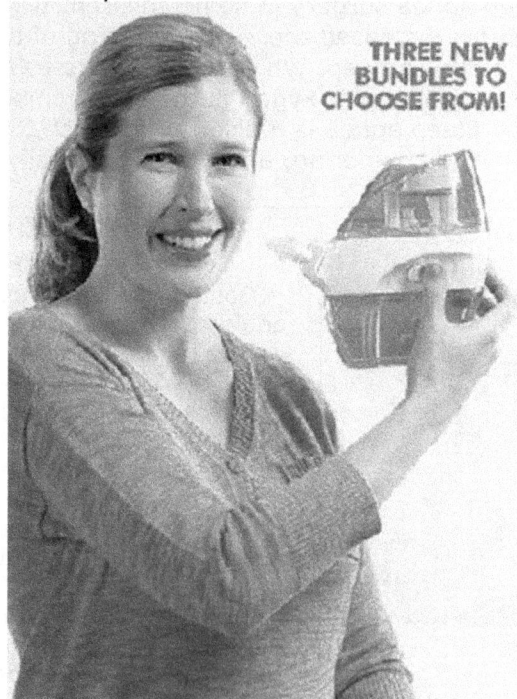

Courtesy of Navage
Figure 6.4 Navage nasal spray unit.

(iv) MyPurMist Handheld Steam Inhaler [8]
www.MyPurMist.com

MyPurMist is designed to deliver direct relief to your nose, sinuses and throat, so you can breathe well and sleep well.

The MyPurMist.com website claims that:
- This device is the World's most advanced steam inhaler - period!
- Provides instant germ-free, allergen-free and pollutant-free therapeutic fine mist that penetrates deep for superb relief
- Cordless and handheld, so that you can use it anywhere, anytime;
  No maintenance needed
- 100% natural and drug-free therapy for sinus congestion, colds and allergies. Steam is recommended by doctors and medical institutions
- Doubles as a HEPA air purifier
- Bluetooth connectivity with mobile app to optimize your results
- Ultrapure Advantage. Combining ultrapure sterile water, our patented CFV instant steam device, and a medical-grade HEPA filter, provides pure therapeutic warm mist - effectively free from germs, allergens, and pollutants
- A Bluetooth processor and the MyPurMist mobile app provide a modern approach to managing upper respiratory conditions naturally, effectively and easily

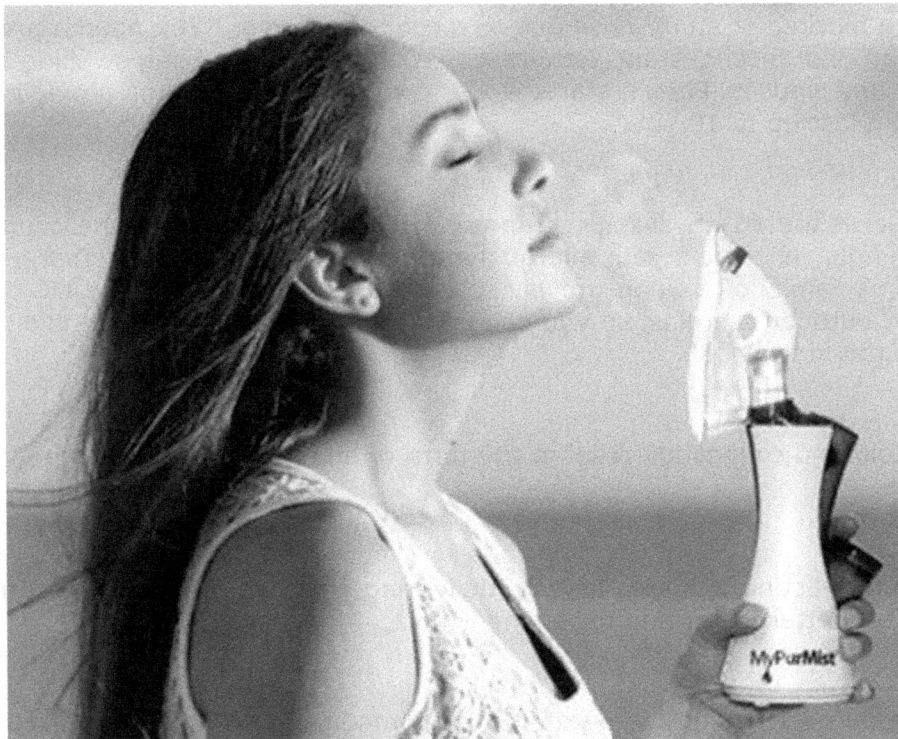

Courtesy of MyPurMist
Figure 6.5 MyPurMist steam inhaler unit.

(iv) Other Nasal Sprays Available at HealthSnap.ca [9]
https://www.healthsnap.ca/category/medicine-cabinet-category/allergy-and-sinus-category/

The Healthsnap.ca website has been advertising the following nasal sprays, nasal creams, inhalers or tablets. Each product has its unique application. The patient has to try the product of his/her choice, by consulting an appropriate healthcare professional to find out if the product is suitable to treat the nasal congestion, sinus infection, allergies or other medical condition such as mild sleep apnea. HealthSnap.ca posted the following descriptions on their website:

1. NeilMed
NeilMed is the largest manufacturer and supplier of LVLP (Large Volume Low Pressure) saline nasal irrigation systems in the world. The NeilMed brand of products help alleviate common nasal and sinus symptoms in a simple, safe, effective and affordable way.

2. HydraSense
HydraSense is the only line of nasal care products sold in Canada and made with 100% undiluted natural-source seawater. HydraSense sources its seawater exclusively from tides in the Bay of Saint-Malo in France. Being one of the most powerful tides in the world, its composition is constantly renewed by the strong currents, oxygenating it and replenishing it of its mineral salt content.

3. Otrivin
Suffering from a blocked or stuffy nose due to a cold or allergies? You need a product like Otrivin. Unlike an oral decongestant, Otrivin works directly by reducing swelling in your nasal passages and sinuses. Plus, it starts working within a few minutes providing relief, and its effect can last up to 10 hours.

4. Claritin
Live Claritin Clear is the #1 physician-recommended, non-drowsy, over-the-counter brand for effective 24-hour relief from your allergy symptoms caused by pollen, dust, mould and pets.The Claritin® family offers non-drowsy solutions that provide fast and effective relief from indoor and outdoor allergies, so you can be alert and focused as if you did not have any allergies in the first place.

5. Dristan
Dristan offers cold and congestion relief in the form of a long-lasting nasal spray and multi-symptom tablets.

6. Drixoral
Drixoral is both fast-acting and long-lasting, delivering effective relief that lasts up to 12 hours, so you feel better faster and for a long time.

7. Reactine
Reactine is Canada's #1 indoor and outdoor allergy medication. For allergy symptom relief, Reactine provides a range of medicinal products to get you back to your day.

8. Rhinaris
Rhinaris Lubricating Nasal Gel helps moisturize and lubricate dry and stuffy noses. It is formulated to provide long-lasting relief from dry nasal passages caused by low humidity environments.

9. SinuCleanse
Established in 1997 by a leading ear, nose and throat physician, SinuCleanse has developed a unique line of revolutionary products for nasal relief, washing the painful symptoms associated with sinus issues experienced by over 70 million Americans. All products manufactured by this brand are 100% safe and natural as well as very effective. Over the years, SinuClease has continued its research and innovation by committing to helping you and your loved ones breathe easier with the power of salt naturally.

10. Little Remedies
Little Remedies products are unique because they contain only what's needed to make your child feel better. That means no dyes, no artificial flavours and no alcohol, ever.

11. Nasacort Allergy 24HR
Nasacort Allergy 24HR is an over-the-counter intranasal steroid (INS) used to treat nasal symptoms for indoor and outdoor allergies (perennial and seasonal allergic rhinitis). When Nasacort is used as directed, it can relieve the symptoms of allergic rhinitis (AR): sneezing, runny nose, nasal itching and congestion. Nasacort is not for children under 2 years of age.

12. Aerius
Aerius is an antihistamine that delivers multi-symptom allergy relief for up to 24 hours. Antihistamines are effective in reducing the symptoms caused by your body's reaction to allergens by blocking the action of histamine, a substance produced by the body in response to allergens like dust and dust mites, pollen from ragweed, grass, trees, or fur from dogs and cats.

13. Vicks
The Vicks legacy is about more than just cold and flu medicine. It's about giving families the opportunity to get more out of life, every day—even on sick days—for more than 100 years. So go ahead: Breathe Life In. Vicks will be there for you.

Obstructive Sleep Apnea in Children and Adolescents [10]

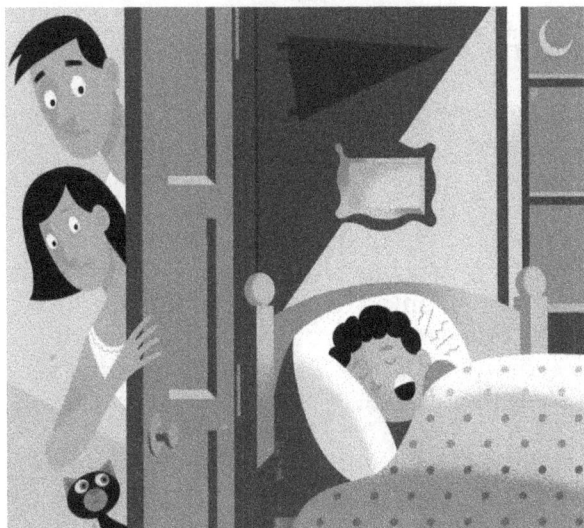

Obstructive sleep apnea in babies, children and adolescents is actually different than the sleep apnea we find and experience in adults. While adults usually have tiredness and daytime sleepiness, children are affected by allergy symptoms such as noisy breathing, sneezing, runny nose with clear mucus, itchy and watery eyes, nasal congestion & sinus pressure. Eventually some children develop snoring, "Obstructive Sleep Apnea (OSA)," and behavioral problems.

Medications such as steroid nasal sprays, saline nasal rinses, and allergy medications, may help relieve mild sleep apnea symptoms. These medications can reduce airway constriction, and poor tongue posture caused by constantly breathing through the mouth.

Figure 6.6 Allergy medications (OTCs) may help relieve mild obstructive sleep apnea.

HOW TO KNOW IF THIS TREATMENT IS WORKING OR NOT?

ANSWER: Take the "overnight pulse oximetry test" before and after the therapy, and compare the results (Desaturation Index and mean SpO2).

If your child has nasal congestion or sinuses, and if the problem is left untreated, it could lead to mild sleep apnea, moderate sleep apnea or even severe sleep apnea.

Most children with nasal congestion are diagnosed with mild sleep apnea. There are also some clinical studies in which the researchers reported that mild sleep apnea in children can be treated with nasal sprays. So it is important that using the nasal spray daily with appropriate care and caution is of utmost importance to treat mild sleep apnea in children. There is no way you could treat moderate or severe sleep apnea with nasal sprays. They simply won't work!

If Your Child Has Mild Obstructive Sleep Apnea, Do the Following:

(i) <u>Take control of your child's health into your own hands</u>. Do not depend on hospitals, doctors, nurses, or CPAP vendors who can do the "overnight pulse oximetry test" for you. Do your own test, and learn how to do it confidently on your own if you want to reverse or improve sleep apnea.

(ii) Purchase and learn how to use the Philips Respironics Pulse Oximeter, or Nonin Pulse Oximeter, ResMed Oximeter, Wrist Pulse Oximeter, or any other pulse oximeter to do "overnight pulse oximetry test." Do not rely on cheap devices (they could generate misleading results, so test the device before using it).

(iii) When you get up in the morning after completing the "overnight pulse oximetry test" for your child, you should plug in your pulse oximeter to the USB-drive of your computer, upload the data from pulse oximeter to your computer. The computer program generates the report, and displays it on your computer screen. You should focus your attention on two important results when reading the report: (i) Desaturation Index (events/hr), and (ii) Mean SpO2 (%).The normal Desaturation Index should be less than 5 events/hr. The normal Mean SpO2 (%) should be more than 95%.

(iv) FIRST NIGHT: Take the "overnight pulse oximetry test" the night just before the therapy, without using any nasal spray treatment. Check the results eagerly looking for the Desaturation Index (events/hr) and Mean SpO2 (%) the next morning. Record these values carefully.

(v) Then start using the nasal spray treatment on your child for 6 weeks.

(vi) After 6 weeks of nasal spray treatment, do the "overnight pulse oximetry test" again. Check the results eagerly looking for the Desaturation Index (events/hr) and Mean SpO2 (%) the next morning. Record these values carefully.

(vii) Then compare the results (before using the nasal spray and after using the nasal spray). If the Desaturation Index and Mean SpO2 have improved after using the nasal spray for 6 weeks, it means the treatment is working, and you should continue the same treatment. If the Desaturation Index and Mean SpO2 have not improved after using the nasal spray for 6 weeks, it means the nasal spray treatment is not working. You should seek another type of nasal spray or other treatment plan to treat the mild sleep apnea of your child.

(viii) If your child's Desaturation Index (events/hr) is under 5, and also if the Mean SpO2 level is over 95% <u>from an "overnight pulse oximetry test," without using any nasal spray,</u> that means your child's sleep apnea is completely reversed.

CHAPTER 6   NASAL SPRAYS

REFERENCES

1. Nasal Sprays for Cold Relief by WebMD.
https://www.webmd.com/cold-and-flu/cold-guide/nasal-sprays-cold-relief#1

2. What Does A Nasal Spray Do? By Huffington Post.
http://www.huffingtonpost.ca/2013/11/14/what-does-nasal-spray-do_n_4275256.html

3. Neti Pot Use: How To Help Sinus Infections Naturally, Rebecca Zamon, The Huffington Post Canada.
http://www.huffingtonpost.ca/2014/03/21/neti-pot-use_n_5000376.html

4. Flonase Nasal Spray.
https://www.flonase.com/
http://www.flonase.ca/

5. Report: Flonase May Combat Sleep Apnea, Posted by Don Amerman in Allergy Relief September 14, 2013.
https://www.accessrx.com/blog/allergy-relief/report-flonase-may-combat-sleep-apnea-m0830/

6. Anti-inflammatory therapy for obstructive sleep apnea in children, Bat-Chen Friedman, MD and Ran D. Goldman, MD FRCPC.
https://www.ncbi.nlm.nih.gov/pmc/articles/PMC3155440/

7. Navage Nose Cleanser Websites.
https://www.navage.com/
https://www.navage.ca/en/

8. MyPurMist Handheld Steam Inhaler.
www.MyPurMist.com

9. Nasal Sprays Available at HealthSnap.ca.
https://www.healthsnap.ca/category/medicine-cabinet-category/allergy-and-sinus-category/

10. Children and Sleep Apnea: What it is, how it harms chilrdrens' sleep and health, and how it can be treated by Sleep Foundation, Updated June 24, 2021.
https://www.sleepfoundation.org/sleep-apnea/children-and-sleep-apnea

CHAPTER 7 SLEEP APNEA TREATMENT Section-V

POSITIONAL THERAPY: SIDE SLEEPING WORKS!

TABLE OF CONTENTS

CHAPTER 7 SLEEP APNEA TREATMENT Section-V

POSITIONAL THERAPY: SIDE SLEEPING WORKS!

British Snoring and Sleep Apnea Association posted the following information: [1]
Body position plays an important role during sleep and can often make the difference between having a good night's sleep or not. For snorers and individuals who suffer from obstructive sleep apnea (OSA), this is a particular problem as several studies have found that individuals who sleep in the supine position (on the back) are more likely to snore or have increased apneas than those who sleep in the lateral position (on the side).

The soft tissue of the throat is likely to collapse and block the airway if you sleep on your back (supine position). Several clinical studies proved that the soft tissue of the throat is less likely to collapse and block the airway if you sleep on your side. Sleep position has a great influence on obstructive sleep apnea and also on many other health conditions. The following are the four common sleep positions: [2]

a. Sleeping On the Left Side: Health experts recommend that the sleeping on your left side is the best habit, not only to treat obstructive sleep apnea but also to protect your overall health. If you suffer from mild obstructive sleep apnea, sleeping on your left side alone might help you treat your disorder. But you should make sure you do not switch to other sleep positions during the sleep.

b. Sleeping On the Back (Supine): Sleeping on the back is not recommended if you have obstructive sleep apnea. The soft tissue easily relaxes, collapses and blocks the airway. It could also cause back pain problems if your bed is not perfectly flat.

c. Sleeping On the Right Side: Again sleeping on the right side is not recommended if you suffer from obstructive sleep apnea because gravity will make it easier for the contents of the stomach to splash back into the upper airway, blocking the inhaled air into the lungs.

d. Sleeping On the Stomach or Chest (Prone): This position again could cause back pain and neck pain problems because of the strain of the musculature around the upper spine and neck vertebrae.

CLINICAL STUDY-I [3, 4]

A clinical study published in 2012 reported that the Positional Obstructive Sleep Apnea (POSA) can be effectively treated by positional therapy, by sleeping on the side throughout the night. In this study, 16 patients who could not tolerate CPAP therapy were tested with positional therapy by using a device that would keep the patients in the side-sleeping position throughout the night for a period of 3 months. The scientists tested their performance by means of an actigraphic recorder. The results for "before wearing the device" and "after wearing it for 3 months" were compared, and it was concluded that positional therapy or side sleeping works, and significantly reduces the sleep apnea. Desaturation Index (events/hour) was found to be decreased.

TENNIS BALL TECHNIQUE FOR SIDE SLEEPING [5, 6]

The tennis ball technique for treating sleep disorders such as snoring and obstructive sleep apnea was introduced in 1980s. In this technique, a tennis ball is fastened on the back of the patient with a belt or strap, so that the patient would feel uncomfortable sleeping on the back, and would instead roll over and sleep on the side, thereby avoiding any collapse of the soft tissue of the throat. This technique could keep the airway open during sleep and could significantly reduce the sleep apnea events per hour.

CLINICAL STUDY-II [5]

A clinical study involving 67 people (aged 60 or over, either obese or overweight) diagnosed with obstructive sleep apnea reported the following: When they were diagnosed with obstructive sleep apnea, their average Desaturation Index was 29.6 events/hour. When the patients were asked to sleep intentionally on their backs, their apnea-hypopnea index (AHI) soared to 53 events/hour. After that they were carefully allowed to sleep on the side by using the tennis ball technique. When the patients slept on the side, their apnea-hypopnea index (AHI) dropped to 14.1 events/hour, indicating that positional therapy cured sleep apnea. The major problem reported by the patients if they used tennis ball technique was that it was very uncomfortable and some patients developed back pain.

PROS & CONS OF THE POSITIONAL THERAPY

As reported in the aforementioned clinical study, positional therapy did not reduce the apnea-hypopnea index (AHI) to less than 5. Whereas the CPAP machine is capable of reducing the apnea-hypopnea index (AHI) to less than 5 every single night and whenever the patient sleeps with the CPAP machine. That means positional therapy is not as effective as the CPAP therapy, but it is a good alternative for those who could not tolerate the use of a CPAP machine accompanied by a mask. By using positional therapy every single night, severe sleep apnea can be reduced to moderate sleep apnea or moderate sleep apnea can reduced to mild sleep apnea, thereby minimizing the high risk associated with the sleep disorder called "sleep apnea."

CLINICAL STUDY-III [7]
Results

Positional Therapy (PT) was used by 53 patients, of which 40 patients underwent a follow-up polygraphic evaluation under treatment, after a median time interval of 12 weeks. Patients were routinely contacted regarding their clinical status and treatment compliance.

Conclusion

PT using the tennis ball technique is an easy method to treat most patients with positional OSA on a short-term basis, showing significant reductions in AHI. Unfortunately, long-term compliance is low and close follow-up of patients on PT with regard to their compliance is necessary.

CLINICAL STUDY-IV [8]

Results : 145 POSA patients were included. 106 patients registered online and uploaded their SPT data to the online database. Compliance, defined as use of the SPT for at least four hours per night, was 64.4%. During the 6 months follow up, the median percentage of supine sleep decreased rapidly after therapy started, and this decrease was stable over time. Median ESS changed from 11 to 7, FOSQ from 91 to 103, PSQI from 7 to 6.

Conclusion: SPT applied for 6 months is a successful and well tolerated treatment for patients with POSA, which diminishes subjective sleepiness, improves sleep-related quality of life and effectively reduces percentage of supine sleep time. Further research, especially in comparing its efficacy to other treatments is ongoing.

POSA=Positional Obstructive Sleep Apnea
STP=Sleep Position Trainer
ESS = Epworth Sleepiness Scale
PSQI = Pittsburgh Sleep Quality Index
FOSQ = Functional Outcome of Sleep Questionnaire

SIDE SLEEPING POSITION KEEPS THE AIRWAY OPEN SO YOU CAN CONTROL YOUR SLEEP APNEA!

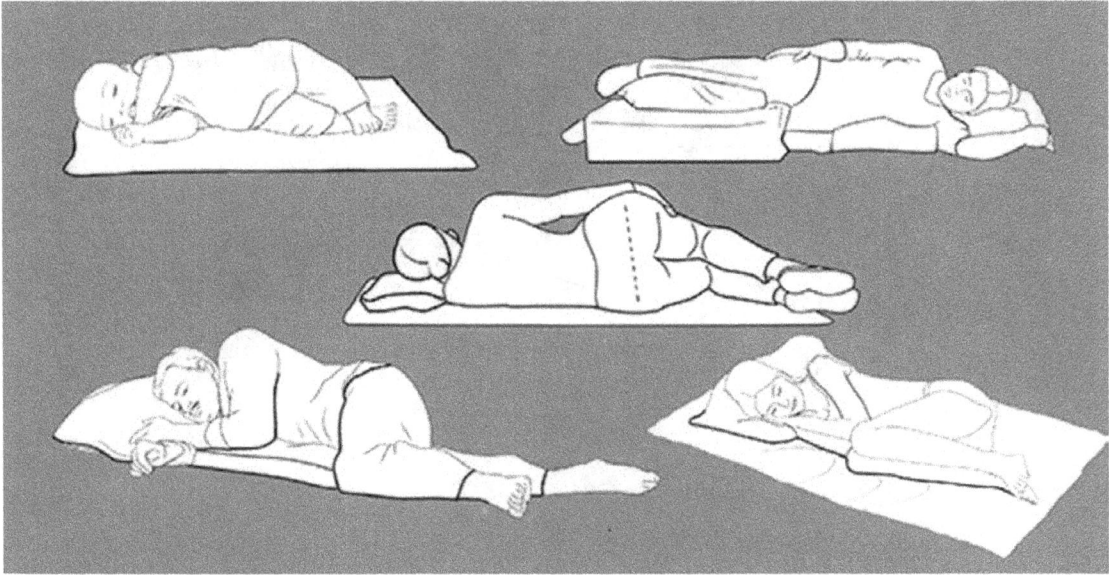

Figure 7.1 Side sleeping positions that help relieve sleep apnea. Side-sleeping opens your airway, improves your breathing, stops snoring, and helps you sleep better.

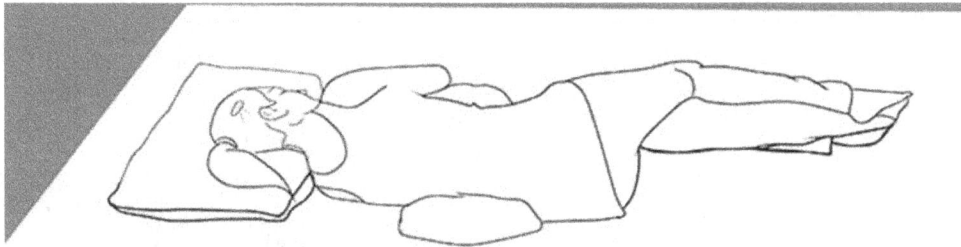

Figure 7.2 Side sleeping positions that help relieve sleep apnea. Side-sleeping opens your airway, improves your breathing, stops snoring, and helps you sleep better.

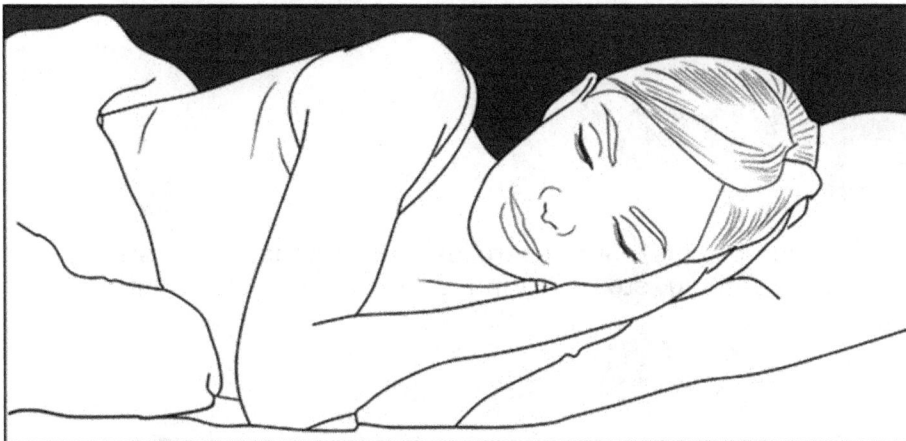

Figure 7.3 Side sleeping position that helps relieve sleep apnea. Side-sleeping opens your airway, improves your breathing, stops snoring, and helps you sleep better.

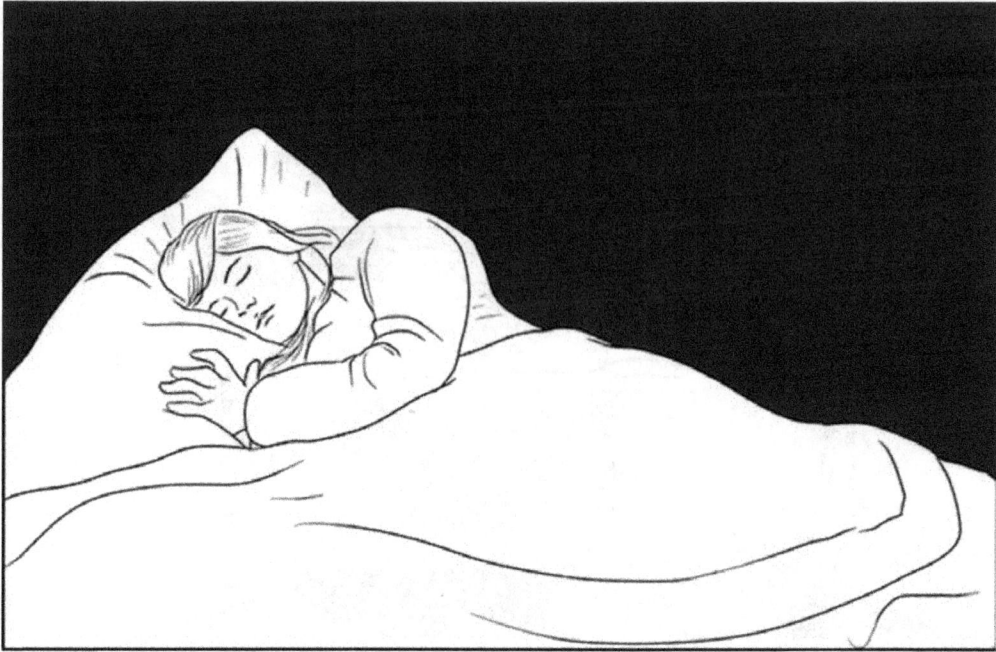

Figure 7.4 Side sleeping position that helps relieve sleep apnea. Side-sleeping opens your airway, improves your breathing, stops snoring, and helps you sleep better.

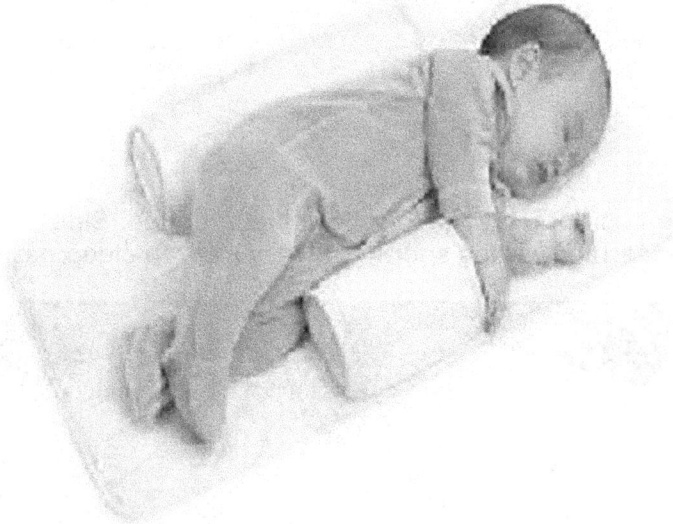

Figure 7.3 Side sleeping position that helps relieve sleep apnea. Side-sleeping opens your airway, improves your breathing, stops snoring, and helps you sleep better.

Side Sleeping Device-I: Zzoma Side Sleeping Belt [9]
Zzoma Belt (The Prescription for Positional Sleep Apnea)
Anti-Snoring Device for Mild Sleep Apnea
http://zzomaosa.com/

Zzoma is an FDA-cleared positional medical device approved for the treatment of sleep apnea. Designed by board-certified sleep physicians, Zzoma has undergone rigorous clinical trials and reviews and is now available by prescription only.

Clinicians who diagnose patients with mild to moderate sleep apnea may prescribe Zzoma as a first line therapy or as an alternative for patients who cannot adjust to CPAP therapy. Patients who struggle to comply with CPAP devices may find Zzoma a more comfortable alternative to wearing a mask.

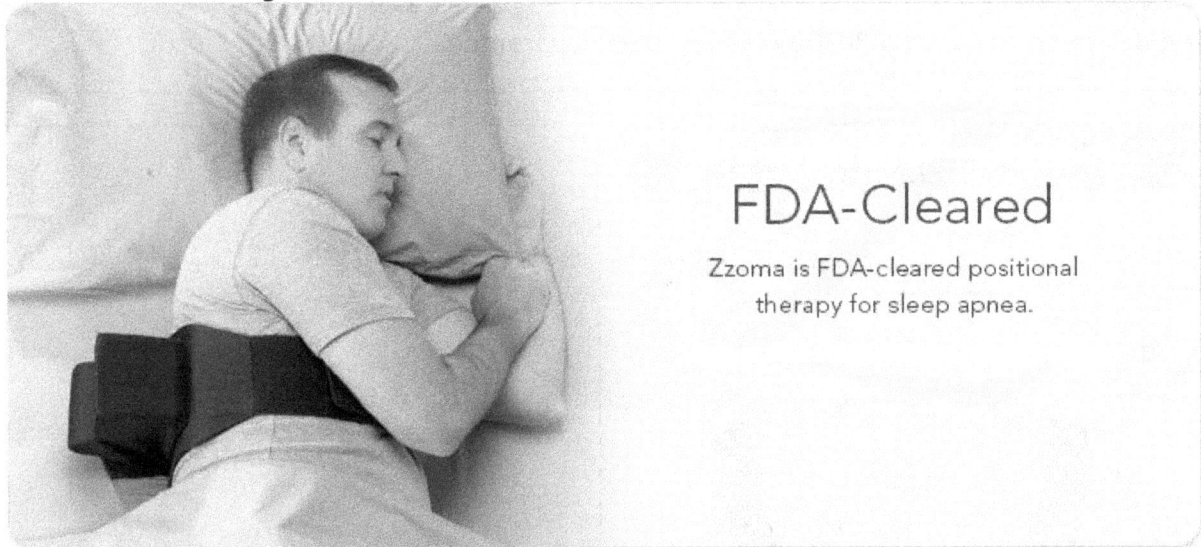

FDA-Cleared

Zzoma is FDA-cleared positional therapy for sleep apnea.

Figure 7.6   Zzoma side-sleeping belt, FDA-cleared (Picture 1).

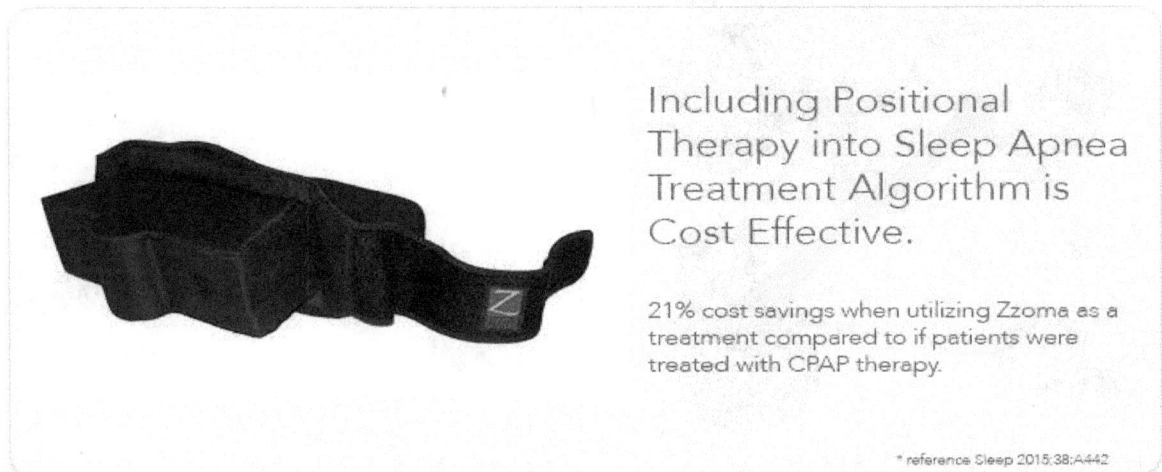

Including Positional Therapy into Sleep Apnea Treatment Algorithm is Cost Effective.

21% cost savings when utilizing Zzoma as a treatment compared to if patients were treated with CPAP therapy.

* reference Sleep 2015;38:A442

Courtesy of Zzomaosa.com
Figure 7.7   Zzoma side-sleeping belt, FDA-cleared (Picture 2).

Side Sleeping Device-II: The Essential Combo Kit [10]
Anti-Snoring Shirt
https://rematee.com/

● Adult Sizes Available: Medium, Large and Extra Large. If your chest measures more than 50", purchase an extension strap for your belt.
● Adjustable Neoprene Bumper Belt comfortably holds you on your side. Wear your belt over any shirt or pajamas, or directly against your skin.
● The inflatable bumpers can easily be adjusted to your preferred comfort, and deflated for compact traveling.
● The adjustable shoulder straps pre-assembled onto the belt keep the belt in place and allow you to wear your belt high and loose.
● The wash/travel pouch protects your machine-washable belt and makes it convenient to carry during travel.
● The device comes with a 30-Day Money-Back Guarantee.

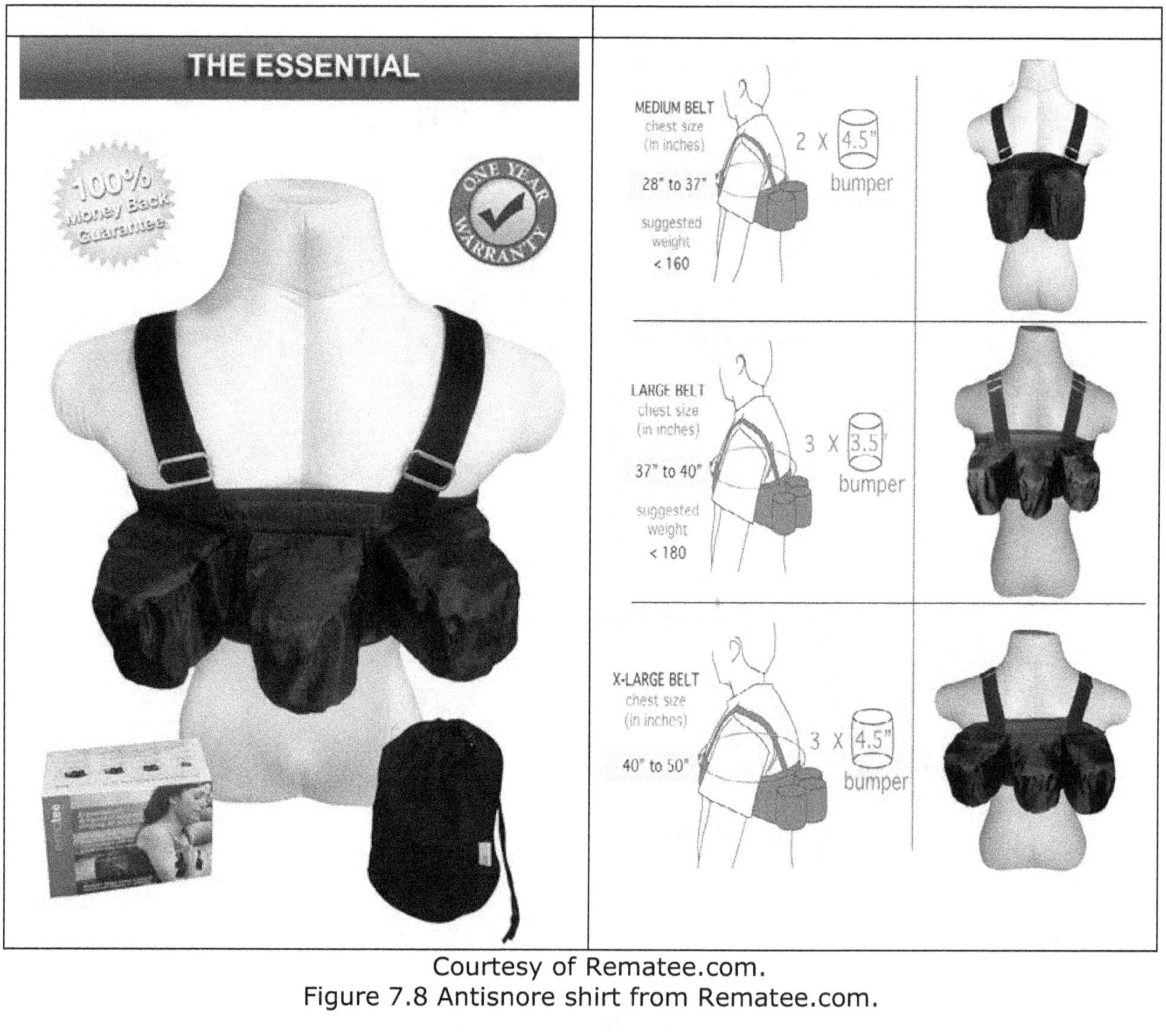

Courtesy of Rematee.com.
Figure 7.8 Antisnore shirt from Rematee.com.

Raise the Head Side of Your Bed Or Use a Thick Pillow [11]

By raising the head side of the bed by as much as 30 to 45 degrees, you can counteract the effects of gravity on blocking the airway. Consider an adjustable bed or simply propping yourself on pillows or a sleeping wedge may be helpful. Sleeping on your left side together with support from pillows to raise your head would allow more inhaled air to enter your lungs.

Take an overnight oximetry test at home to check if this sleeping position improves the Desaturation Index (events/hr) and Mean SpO2 level.

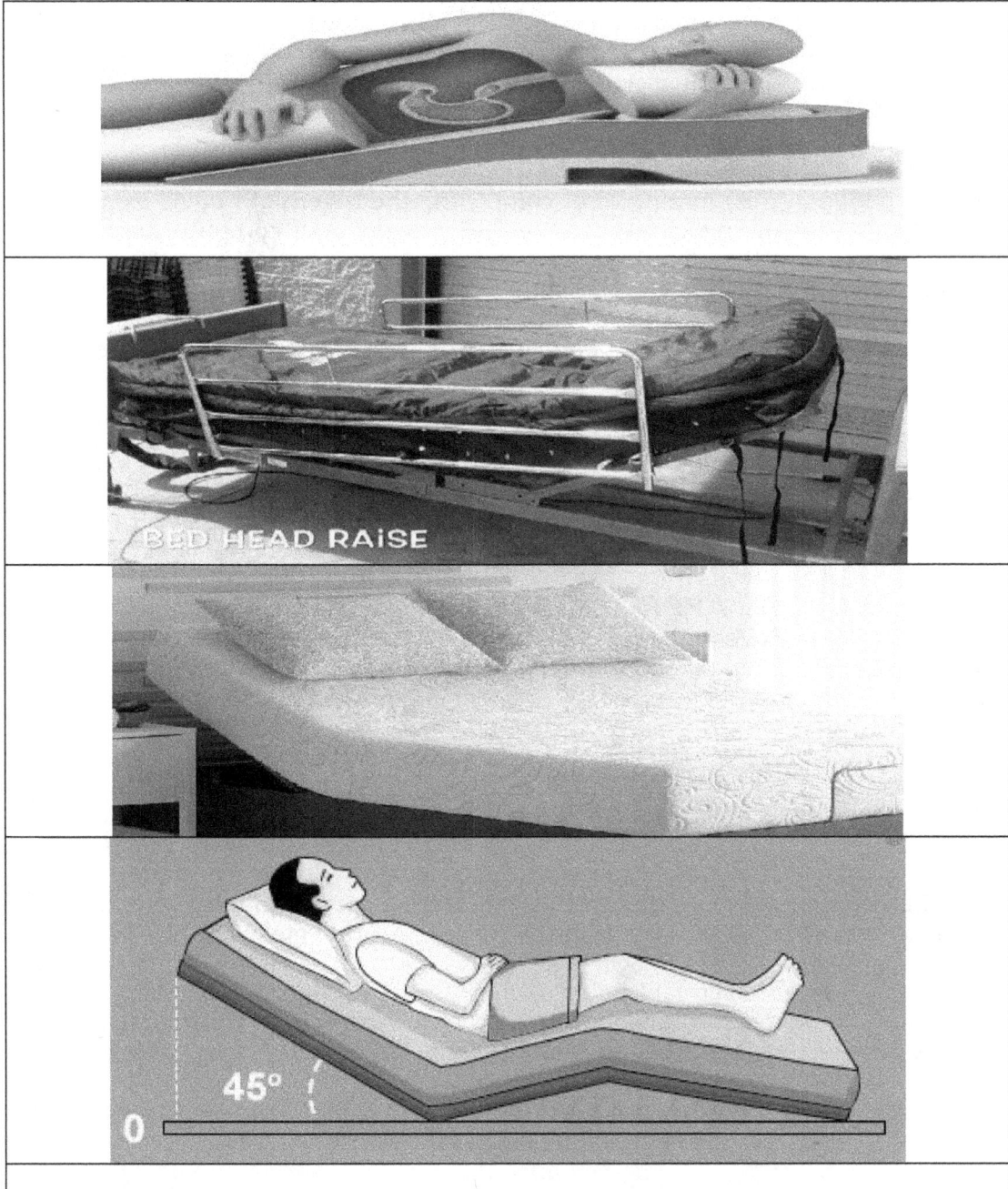

Figure 7.9 Pictures showing "raise the head side of your bed."

HOW TO KNOW IF THIS TREATMENT IS WORKING OR NOT?

ANSWER: Take the "overnight pulse oximetry test" before and after the therapy, and compare the results (Desaturation Index and mean SpO2).

(i) <u>Take control of your health into your own hands</u>. Do not depend on hospitals, doctors, nurses, or CPAP vendors who can do the "overnight pulse oximetry test" for you. Do your own test, and learn how to do it confidently on your own if you want to reverse or improve your sleep apnea.

(ii) Purchase and learn how to use the Philips Respironics Pulse Oximeter, or Nonin Pulse Oximeter, ResMed Oximeter, Wrist Pulse Oximeter, or any other pulse oximeter to do "overnight pulse oximetry test." Do not rely on cheap devices (they could generate misleading results, so test the device before using it).

(iii) When you get up in the morning after completing the "overnight pulse oximetry test," you should plug in your pulse oximeter to the USB-drive of your computer, upload the data from pulse oximeter to your computer. The computer program generates the report, and displays it on your computer screen. You should focus your attention on two important results when reading the report: Desaturation Index (events/hr), and Mean SpO2 (%). The normal Desaturation Index should be less than 5 events/hr. The normal Mean SpO2 (%) should be more than 95%.

(iv) If the Desaturation Index (events/hr) and Mean SpO2 (%) of the current test are better than the most recent test and all the preceding tests, that means your sleep apnea is improved. If these results are worse than those of all the preceding tests, that means your sleep apnea has worsened. You should take appropriate steps (switch to another therapy or lose your excess body weight) to improve your results (i) Desaturation Index (events/hr), and (ii) Mean SpO2 (%).

HOW TO SELECT THE APPROPRIATE POSITIONAL THERAPY DEVICE?

(i) 1st NIGHT: Take the "overnight pulse oximetry test" without using any therapy or any device. Early in the morning, upload the data from oximeter to your computer, and record the results such as Desaturation Index (events/hr) and Mean SpO2 (%).

(ii) 2nd NIGHT: Take the "overnight pulse oximetry test" by sleeping on your side without using any device. Early in the morning, upload the data from oximeter to your computer, and record the results such as Desaturation Index (events/hr) and Mean SpO2 (%).

(iii) 3rd NIGHT: Take the "overnight pulse oximetry test" by sleeping on your side using device # 1. Early in the morning, upload the data from oximeter to your computer, and record the results such as Desaturation Index (events/hr) and Mean SpO2 (%).

(iv) 4th NIGHT: Take the "overnight pulse oximetry test" by sleeping on your side using device # 2. Early in the morning, upload the data from oximeter to your computer, and record the results such as Desaturation Index (events/hr) and Mean SpO2 (%).

(v) Compare the results (Desaturation Index and Mean SpO2) of all the aforementioned tests. Choose a device that gave you the best Desaturation Index (lowest), and the best SpO2 level (highest).

(vi) Continue your positional therapy with the device that gave you the best Desaturation Index, and the best SpO2 level.

CHAPTER 7 SLEEP APNEA TREATMENT Section-V

REFERENCES

1. Sleeping Position by British Snoring and Sleep Apnea Association.
https://www.britishsnoring.co.uk/why_do_i_snore/sleeping_position.php

2. Sleeping Positions, OSA and CPAP by Tamara Kaye Sellman RPSGT CCSH, March 19, 2017.
https://www.sleepresolutions.com/blog/sleeping-positions-osa-and-cpap-rem-related-osa-and-sleeping-supine

3. Positional Therapy for Sleep Apnea, Sleep Apnea Guide.
http://www.sleep-apnea-guide.com/positional-therapy.html

4. Clinical Study: Positional therapy for obstructive sleep apnea: an objective measurement of patients' usage and efficacy at home. Authors: Heinzer RC1, Pellaton C, Rey V, Rossetti AO, Lecciso G, Haba-Rubio J, Tafti M, Lavigne G.
https://www.ncbi.nlm.nih.gov/pubmed/22261242

5. Positional Therapy: Sleep Apnea & The Tennis Ball Technique by Sleep Education Blog
http://sleepeducation.blogspot.ca/2009/10/positional-therapy-sleep-apnea-tennis.html

6. Sticking with the Position by C. A. Wolski Published on May 26, 2015.
http://www.sleepreviewmag.com/2015/05/sticking-position/

7. Clinical Study: Usage of Positional Therapy in Adults with Obstructive Sleep Apnea
Grietje E. de Vries, MSc1,2; Aarnoud Hoekema, MD, PhD; Michiel H.J. Doff, DMD, PhD3; Huib A.M. Kerstjens, MD, PhD1,2; Petra M. Meijer, NP1,4; Johannes H. van der Hoeven, MD, PhD5; Peter J. Wijkstra, MD, PhD1,2,4.
http://www.aasmnet.org/jcsm/ViewAbstract.aspx?pid=29877
http://dx.doi.org/10.5664/jcsm.4458

8. Clinical Study: Sleep Position Trainer vs.Tennis Ball Technique in Positional Obstructive Sleep Apnoea Syndrome.
http://www.nightbalance.com/email/Combi%20Eijsvogel,%20van%20Maanen,%20van%20Maanen.pdf

9. Zzoma Belt: The Prescription for Positional Sleep Apnea.
http://zzomaosa.com/

10. Rematee Side Sleeping Device, Rematee, 1124 Fir Ave, Blaine, WA 98230, USA.
https://rematee.com/

11. Snoring Treatment Options: 16 Remedies to Stop Snoring Tonight, Health & Fitness, 16 May 2015 14:24 CET.
https://www.modernghana.com/lifestyle/7977/16/snoring-treatment-options-16-remedies-to-s.html

CHAPTER 8 SLEEP APNEA TREATMENT Section-VI

NATURAL THERAPY: LIFESTYLE CHANGES

TABLE OF CONTENTS

CHAPTER 8 SLEEP APNEA TREATMENT Section-VI

NATURAL THERAPY: LIFESTYLE CHANGES

Table 8.1 Natural therapy to relieve and even reverse obstructive sleep apnea.

The following natural therapy may help you relieve and even reverse your obstructive sleep apnea:	
1	**Quit Smoking**
2	**Quit Alcohol Consumption**
3	**Train Yourself to Sleep On Your Side** Side-Sleeping Keeps Your Airway Open!
4	**Lose Your Excess Body Weight** **Until Your BMI Drops to Normal** Weight Loss Reverses Sleep Apnea!

QUIT SMOKING IF YOU HAVE SLEEP APNEA [1, 2]

Research showed that smokers are three times more prone to suffering from sleep apnea as compared to non-smokers. Smoking increases inflammation and fluid retention in the upper airway, thereby blocking the inhaled air flow into the lungs. As a result, the SpO2 level goes down during sleep. Research also showed that the sleep apneics who smoke regularly have higher chances of developing cancer, and have heightened triglyceride levels and lowered HDL levels, indicating higher chances of heart disease.

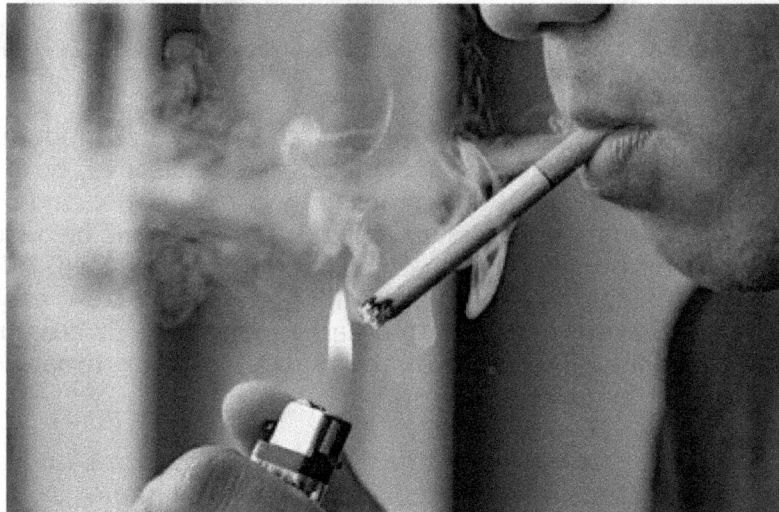

Figure 8.1 Smoking is not only harmful to your general health, but also intensifies sleep apnea.

Continuous smoking (chainsmoking) causes swelling and inflammation in the upper airway of your throat, which in turn blocks the inhaled air causing the SpO2 levels to fall. The combination of smoking and obstructive sleep apnea could create a deadly condition that could wreck your quality of life and could severely shorten your life span.

Before starting any sleep apnea treatment, the sleep apneics must go through the process of quitting smoking (rehab to quit smoking). The patient who tries to quit smoking further faces a nuisance of withdrawal symptoms such as nausea, cramps, headaches, sweating, and even lucid dreaming. It is therefore strongly advised that if you are diagnosed with obstructive sleep apnea or any other type of sleep disorder, you must learn to quit smoking immediately. Otherwise smoking would further complicate your sleep disorder.

QUIT ALCOHOL CONSUMPTION IF YOU HAVE SLEEP APNEA [3, 4, 5, 6, 7, 8]

Avoid alcohol, tranquilizers and sleeping pills. Alcohol consumption relaxes the soft tissue of the muscles in the back of your throat, which makes it collapse easily, thereby blocking the airway when you fall asleep. As a result, the SpO2 level goes down during sleep.

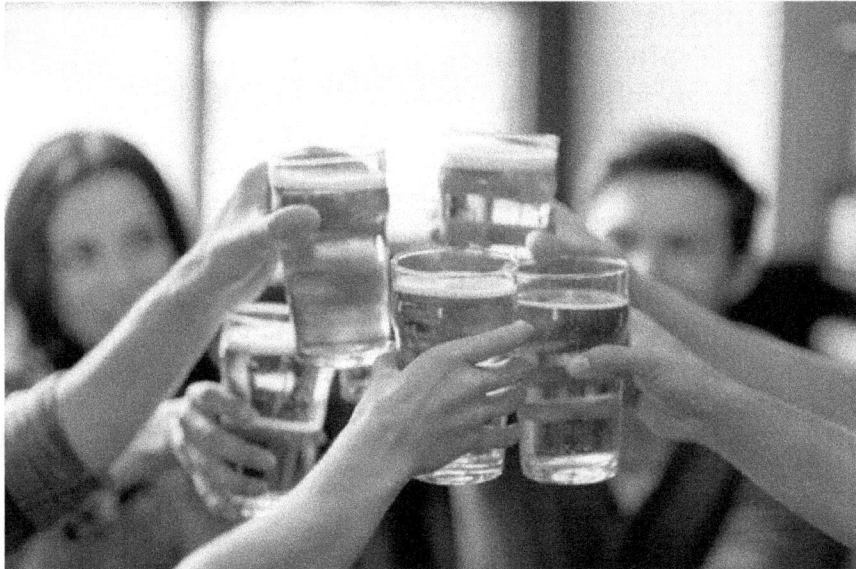

Figure 8.2 Alcohol consumption not only ruins your heart and liver, but also intensifies sleep apnea.

Alcohol makes obstructive sleep apnea worse. Research shows that moderate or heavy drinking of alcohol would increase the length of sleep apnea episodes, both apneas and hypopneas. It means alcohol consumption increases the Desaturation Index and causes the SpO2 levels to fall below normal during sleep. If the SpO2 level falls below dramatically, a person can suffocate himself/herself, and death occurs during the sleep. Additionally, if you are addicted to alcohol, you may be at a higher risk of developing OSA, especially if you already snore. Alcohol decreases your drive to breathe, slowing your breathing and making your breaths shallow. In addition, it may relax the muscles of your throat, which may make it more likely for your upper airway to collapse.

So it is highly recommended that you do not consume alcohol several hours before bedtime in order to minimize the effects overnight. Reduce your alcohol intake. As alcohol, being a stimulant and sedative plays a role in relaxing and collapsing the soft tissue of the throat muscle, thereby causing the obstruction while inhaling and exhaling air into and from the lungs. In addition, alcohol is called a muscle relaxant. It causes the tissues of the throat to relax as well. This can contribute to the risk of both, snoring and sleep apnea. Therefore, it is recommended that you avoid consuming alcohol several hours before bedtime or never drink alcohol if you have obstructive sleep apnea. Quitting alcohol completely would save your life in all respects.

SIDE SLEEPING: TRAIN YOURSELF HOW TO SLEEP ON YOUR SIDE

Stop sleeping on your back, which leads to snoring. Train yourself to sleep on your side, or purchase a device that keeps you on side-sleeping position when you sleep (Please refer to Chapter 7). You will immediately notice that you are not snoring anymore as side-sleeping keeps your airway open. Research showed that side sleeping keeps your airway open (Please refer to Chapter 7). If your airway is open while sleeping, your SpO2 level remain normal over 95%. If your SpO2 is normal, your Desaturation Index (events per hour) would automatically be normal. Which means your sleep apnea is reversed.

LOSE YOUR EXCESS BODY WEIGHT

Scientific research with several randomized studies showed that weight loss reverses obstructive sleep apnea. Learn how to monitor your body mass index (BMI) or body fat percentage (%), and monitor at least once every week. Learn how to eat whole foods only by avoiding the processed foods and refined foods. If you exercise high self-discipline and high will power, it is indeed possible to lose all your excess body weight until your BMI reaches normal value. Research showed that if your BMI is normal, your Desaturation Index (events per hour) would automatically be normal. If the Desturation Index (events per hour) is normal, your Mean SpO2 (%) would automatically be normal. If your Desatiration Index is under 5 events per hour, and if your mean SpO2 and minimum SpO2 are over 95%, that means your obstruction sleep apnea is completely reversed.

HOW TO KNOW IF NATURAL TREATMENT IS HELPING OR NOT?
How To Know if Your Sleep Apnea Is Improved or Worsened?

ANSWER: Take the "overnight pulse oximetry test" before and after the therapy, and compare the results (Desaturation Index and mean SpO2).

(i) Take control of your health into your own hands. Do not depend on hospitals, doctors, nurses, or CPAP vendors who can do the "overnight pulse oximetry test" for you. Do your own test, and learn how to do it confidently on your own if you want to reverse or improve your sleep apnea.

(ii) Purchase and learn how to use the Philips Respironics Pulse Oximeter, or Nonin Pulse Oximeter, ResMed Oximeter, Wrist Pulse Oximeter, or any other pulse oximeter to do "overnight pulse oximetry test." Do not rely on cheap devices (they could generate misleading results, so test the device before using it).

(iii) When you get up in the morning after completing the "overnight pulse oximetry test," you should plug in your pulse oximeter to the USB-drive of your computer, upload the data from pulse oximeter to your computer. The computer program generates the report, and displays results of your test on your computer screen. You should focus your attention on two important results when reading the report: (i) Desaturation Index (events/hr), and (ii) Mean SpO2 (%). The normal Desaturation Index should be less than 5 events/hr. The normal Mean SpO2 (%) should be more than 95%.

(iv) If the Desaturation Index (events/hr) and Mean SpO2 (%) of the current test are better than the most recent test and all the preceding tests, that means your sleep apnea is improved.

(v) If the Desaturation Index (events/hr) and Mean SpO2 (%) of the current test are worse than those of all the preceding tests, that means your sleep apnea has worsened, indicating that the CPAP Therapy is not working. You should take appropriate steps to improve your results. Either switch to another therapy or lose your excess body weight so that your results and therefore your sleep apnea will be improved.

(vi) <u>If your Desaturation Index (events/hr) is under 5, and also if your Mean SpO2 level and minimum SpO2 are over 95% from the most recent test, that means your sleep apnea is completely reversed</u>.

FURTHER GUIDANCE

● Even some 10 to 20 pounds of weight loss would have a significant impact on your obstructive sleep apnea progress. The number of sleep apnea events per hour, what is known as Desaturation Index, during your sleep would significantly decline and the wide fluctuations of SpO2 would stabilize, switching you from severe sleep apnea to moderate sleep apnea, or from moderate sleep apnea to mild sleep apnea, and allowing you to feel a lot better than you have ever felt since your diagnosis.

● You don't have to fully or perfectly reverse your obstructive sleep apnea! If you could manage to switch your Desaturation Index from severe to moderate, or from moderate to mild, that would still be a great accomplishment. Try it out and improve your Desaturation Index (Number of sleep apnea events per hour during the sleep), you will feel a lot better and your overall health improves!

● With determination and steadfastness, you can not only improve your condition or sleep disorder, but also strengthen your ability to respond to your body's functionality and lead a much better life. You should always remember that knowledge is the power, so you must equip your mind with a deep understanding of sleep apnea by collecting as much information as possible, and by reading and researching a lot. Get ready to lower your Desaturation Index and the wide fluctuations of SpO2 during the sleep.

● Your biggest decision is your commitment to setting goals and objectives, focusing on your goal and staying focused until you fully manifest your goal. Motivation, commitment, a strong desire to succeed, high self-discipline and high willpower are the essential qualities you need to implement on yourself to be successful. By awakening the giant within yourself, you can become a sleep apnea guru.

CHAPTER 8 SLEEP APNEA TREATMENT Section-VI
NATURAL THERAPY: LIFESTYLE CHANGES

REFERENCES

1. Sleep Apneics Who Smoke – How Treating Both Conditions Is A Must Do for True Success by Dr. Kevin Berry, July 1, 2011.
https://www.tmjtherapyandsleepcenter.com/sleep-apnea-smoking/

2. The smoking and sleep apnea equation. 1 + 1 = 1,000.
http://join.sleepgroupsolutions.com/nicotine-and-sleep/

3. Snoring, Authored by Dr Oliver Starr, 18 Oct 2017.
https://patient.info/health/snoring-leaflet

4. How Alcohol Affects Sleep Apnea, Dr. Peters Explains Why Alcohol & Sleep Apnea Don't Mix.
https://www.verywell.com/how-alcohol-affects-sleep-apnea-3014680

5. Snoring Treatment Options: 16 Remedies to Stop Snoring Tonight, Health & Fitness, 16 May 2015 14:24 CET.
https://www.modernghana.com/lifestyle/7977/16/snoring-treatment-options-16-remedies-to-s.html

6. How Alcohol Affects Sleep Apnea and Snoring by Relaxing Airway Muscles by Brandon Peters, MD, Medically reviewed by Chris Vincent, MD, Posted on May 25, 2020.
https://www.verywellhealth.com/how-alcohol-affects-sleep-apnea-3014680

7. Alcohol and health: alcohol and sleep by Alberta Health Services, PDF File, 2014.
https://www.albertahealthservices.ca/assets/info/amh/if-amh-alcohol-and-sleep.pdf

8. Alcohol and sleep by sleep foundation, Posted on September 4, 2020.
https://www.sleepfoundation.org/nutrition/alcohol-and-sleep

CHAPTER 9 SLEEP APNEA TREATMENT Section-VI
SURGICAL PROCEDURES

TABLE OF CONTENTS

CHAPTER 9 SLEEP APNEA TREATMENT Section-VII
SURGICAL PROCEDURES

Obstructive Sleep Apnea in Children and Adolescents [1, 2, 3, 4, 5]

Pediatric obstructive sleep apnea in babies, children and adolescents is actually different than the sleep apnea we find and experience in adults. While adults usually have tiredness and daytime sleepiness, children are more likely to have behavioral problems, noisy breathing and snoring. The underlying cause in adults is often obesity, while in children the most common underlying condition is enlargement of the tonsils and adenoids.

If your child has any of the following symptoms, you should immediately consult a pediatric physician, and have your child properly checked and diagnosed with the obstructive sleep apnea, and then seek the appropriate treatment or procedure from a sleep specialist.

Sleep Apnea Symptoms in Children and Adolescents

♦ Noisy breathing, hyperactivity, snoring, mouth breathing, coughing, headaches,
♦ Upper airway infections, trouble falling asleep at night, cessation of breathing,
♦ Restlessness, nightmares, strange sleeping positions, sweating in sleep, teeth grinding,
♦ Obesity, chronic nose running, bedwetting, frequent wakings at night, early rising,
♦ Poor performance in school, difficulty concentrating, failure to thrive.

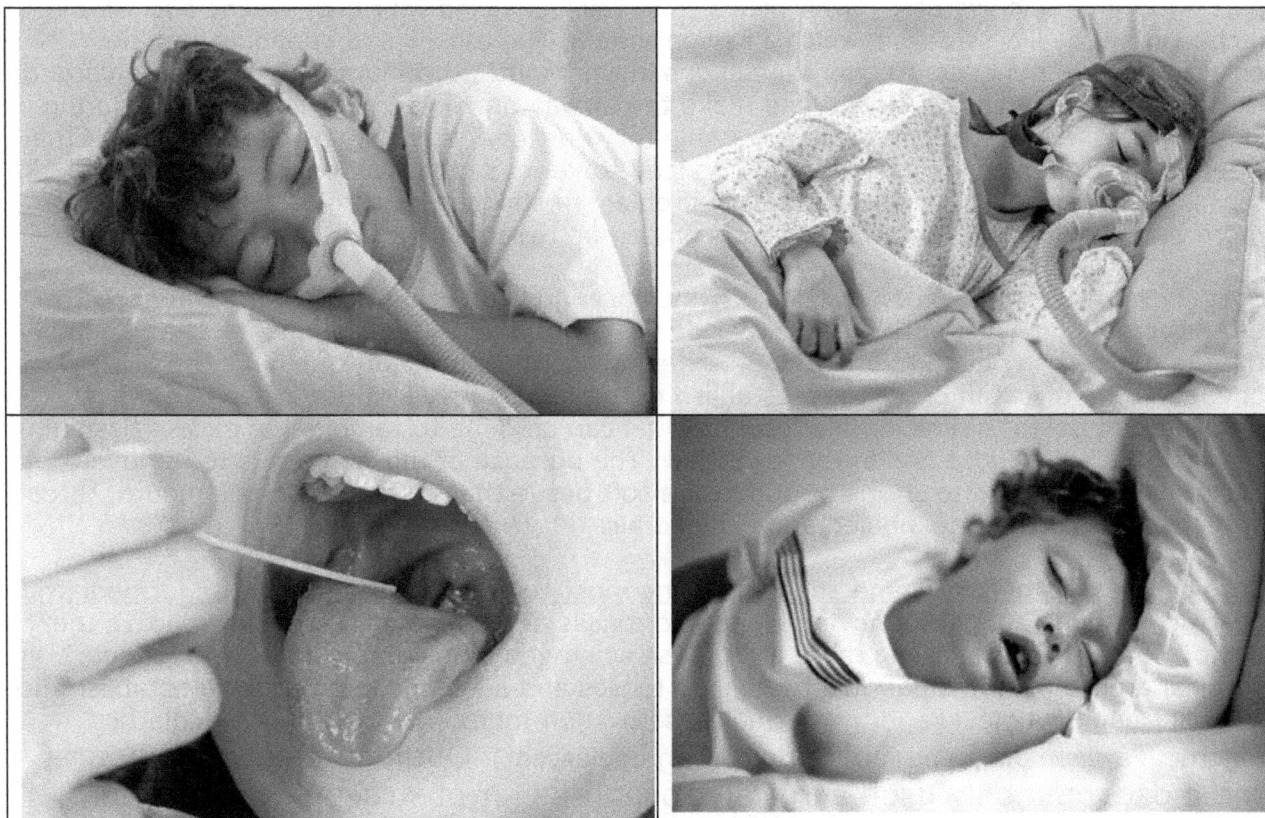

Figure 9. 1 Obstructive sleep apnea in children.

Clinical Diagnosis of Obstructive Sleep Apnea

If your child is experiencing and suffering from the aforementioned symptoms of pediatric obstructive sleep apnea, you should immediately take action and seek a therapy or surgery. After a thorough physical examination, the physician (preferably a sleep clinic specialist) may order either one or both of the following sleep tests:

(i) "Overnight Pulse Oximetry Test" to be performed at home
(ii) "Polysomnogram Test" to be performed in a hospital

Polysomnogram test would be unnecessary in most cases if the results "Desaturation Index (events per hour), Minimum SpO2, Mean SpO2, Mean SpO2 & SpO2 Versus Time Chart" from the "overnight pulse oximetry test" are reliable and trustworthy.

Pediatric obstructive sleep apnea is a sleep disorder in which your child's airway is partially or fully blocked repeatedly during sleep, causing noisy breathing, mouth breathing and snoring. This condition develops due to obstructed nasal airway, poor muscle tone in the throat and tongue, bulky throat tissue, underlined enlarged tonsils and adenoids, long soft palate and/or uvula, and unusually shaped mouth or small mouth.

A widely recognized risk factor for childhood obstructive sleep apnea is enlarged tonsils and adenoids. A lot of children have enlarged tonsils or adenoids (it is a serious problem). Tonsils and adenoids are glands (balls of tissue) located at the back of the throat and are part of the immune system. Tonsils play a small role in helping your body defend against and recover from the illnesses from which a person suffers. The tonsils and adenoids may be enlarged due to genetics, frequent infections in the mouth, or inflammation. When enlarged, these glands constrict the airway and make the airway narrower, making breathing during sleep more difficult, and even stop breathing for short periods of time while sleeping. If their sleep is affected over the long term, it can lead to various complications. Enlargement of tonsils and adenoids is the most common problem in children by surgically removing which more than 90% of the sleep apnea condition can be reversed.

Surgery must be the last resort if the airway blockage is an issue deep in the throat. If the CPAP therapy does not work, and neither do the other alternative treatments, then and only then, a patient may have to undergo an extensive surgical procedure to have the airway opened in the throat in order to re-establish normal SpO2 levels during sleep. A surgical procedure at doctor's clinic or in a local hospital can be done to remove the excess tissue in the mouth, throat, nose and in the lower jaw. The purpose of this surgery is to remove the excess soft tissue and to shrink or stiffen the soft tissue that is hanging in the mouth, throat and nose obstructing the inhaled and exhaled air.

Surgical removal of tonsils and adenoids is the most commonly used procedure for pediatric obstructive sleep apnea. Removing elongated tonsils and adenoids could also improve the airway in the throat, allowing more air to pass when you inhale and exhale. With simple surgical procedures, it is possible to remove tonsils and adenoids in order to re-establish the normal Mean SpO2 level and the normal Desaturation Index (events/hr) of a pediatric obstructive sleep apnea patient (a child or an adolescent). Outlined below briefly are the most commonly used surgical procedures for obstructive sleep apnea.

(i) Tonsils, Adenoids, Tonsillectomy and Adenoidectomy [6, 7]

Swollen tonsils and adenoids block the passage of air in the airway when people inhale and exhale air, and cause obstructive sleep apnea. Tonsillectomy and adenoidectomy are the surgeries being used to remove the tonsils or adenoids mostly in children and in some adults as well. The purpose of the surgery is specifically to treat and relieve obstructive sleep apnea. The surgery requires general anestesia, and a stay of one to few days in the hospital is required. **Before the surgery, the patient should refrain from taking aspirin or other blood thinners, which may cause bleeding during and after the surgery.** A trained and certified surgeon surgically removes the enlarged or excess portion of tissue from the tonsils and adenoids.

AFTER THE SURGERY: The throat will be sore after surgery but pain medications would help. You may find it hard to eat and swallow for a few days so consuming soft and cold fluids are recommended. Some people may experience infection and severe bleeding immediately after the surgery, and these problems can be prevented by prescribing the suitable antibiotics and pain medications. After the surgery, the patient becomes free of the obstructive Sseep apnea (some patients may not be completely free from slep apnea, and may further suffer from mild sleep apnea). An "overnight pulse oximetry test" would reveal that the obstructive sleep apnea is reversed. Desaturation Index would be normal (under 5 events per hour), and the Mean SpO2 would be normal (over 95%).

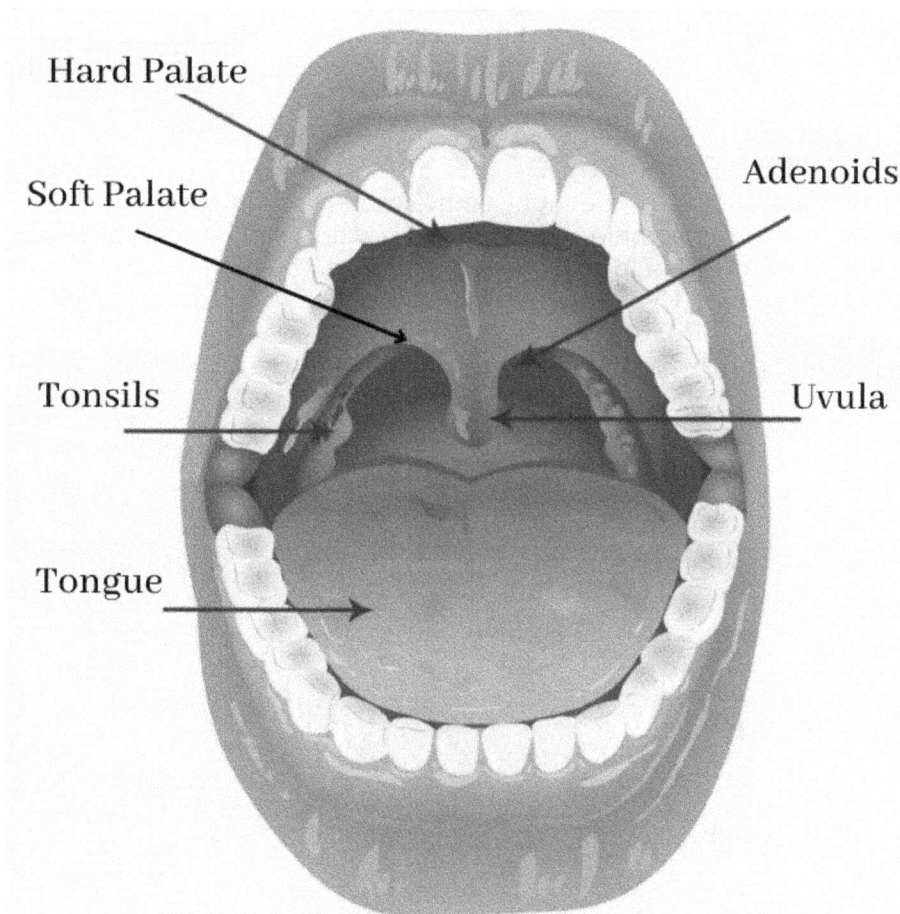

Figure 9.2 Surgery to remove the tonsils or adenoids.

(ii) UPPP (Uvulopalatopharyngoplasty) for Obstructive Sleep Apnea [8, 9]

The soft finger-shaped tissue that hangs down from the back of the roof of the mouth into the throat is called "uvula."

In the Uvulopalatopharyngoplasty (UPPP) procedure, the surgeon removes the excess tissue in the throat to make the airway wider so that more inhaled air passes into the lungs, thus reducing or curing obstructive sleep apnea. In this procedure, the surgeon may remove (i) uvula, (ii) part of the roof of the mouth (soft palate), (iii) excess throat tissue, (iv) tonsils and (v) adenoids.

For most children, removing the tonsils and adenoids (which is a very simple procedure with local anesthesia) could remove the obstruction in the throat and could help re-establish normal breathing, and also cures sleep apnea. If an enlarged tongue is the factor causing obstructive sleep apnea, the surgeon may remove a small part of the tongue. This is called an uvulopalatopharyngoglossoplasty. For some people the Uvulopalatopharyngoplasty (UPPP) procedure may not help re-establish normal breathing, and may not cure sleep apnea completely. In that case, they need to use the CPAP therapy even after surgery.

Laser-assisted removal has gained popularity due to the fact that it can be done as an outpatient or in-office procedure. There is excessive pain involved with the laser procedure as well as the possibility of recurring treatments. Laser-assisted uvulopalatoplasty is not recommended by the American Academy of Sleep Medicine to treat sleep apnea because of further complications.

COMPLICATIONS AFTER SURGERY: Some people may experience complications after surgery such as: bleeding, infection, pain, swelling, problem in swallowing food, inability to speak fluently, insomnia, inability to breath normally, and others. In these cases, some pain medications could help. Watch the following YouTube Video: Uvulopalatopharyngoplasty (UPPP)- Lateral Expansion Pharyngoplasty Variant with Uvulopalatal Flap, May 27, 2020. [10]
https://www.youtube.com/watch?v=D_UNuOdFbMA

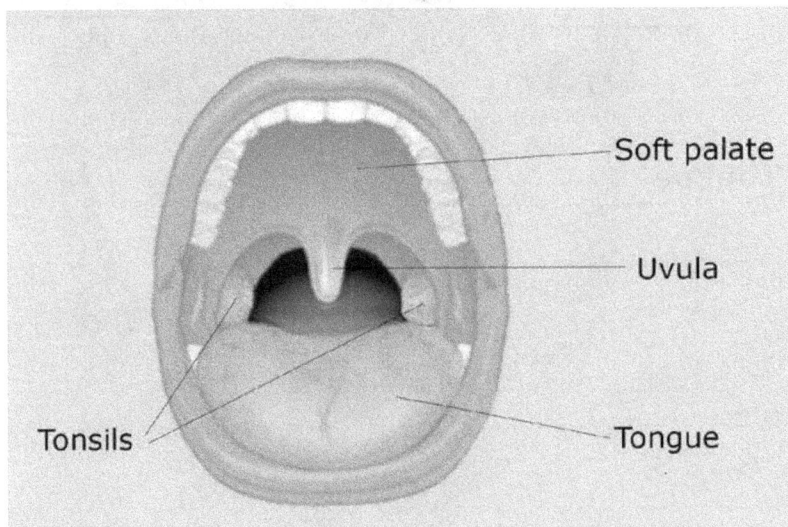

Figure 9.3 Uvulopalatopharyngoplasty (UPPP) procedure.

(iii) THE PILLAR PROCEDURE: Soft Palate Implants [11, 12]

The Pillar® Procedure has long been used to relieve snoring and symptoms of mild to moderate obstructive sleep apnea. The Pillar® Procedure is a simple, safe and effective treatment designed mostly to help you stop severe snoring. It involves the implantation of artificial stabilizers (they could be woven implants or small polyester rods) in the soft palate on the roof of the mouth where the uvula is located, as shown in the picture below. The Pillar Procedure stiffens the soft palate, which is believed to be a significant contributor for at least 80% of patients who could not stop snoring. The Pillar® Procedure can be performed in about 20 minutes, using only local anesthetic and so you can quickly go home and relax on the same day.

The Pillar® Procedure is not recommended for people who have severe obstructive sleep apnea, and to people who are significantly overweight or obese.

The Pillar® Procedure involves surgically placing small polyester rods in the soft palate. Each implant measures 18 mm in length and 1.5 mm in diameter. The subsequent healing of tissue around the implants stiffens the soft palate, thereby reducing relaxation and vibration of the tissue.

In the Pillar® Procedure, a specially trained doctor places tiny woven implants (or small polyester rods) into the soft palate using a sterile delivery tool. Over time, the implants together with the body's natural fibrotic response, add structural support to stiffen the soft palate and reduce the tissue vibration that causes snoring. The implants also stop the tissue from collapsing and obstructing the upper airway thereby causing obstructive sleep apnea.

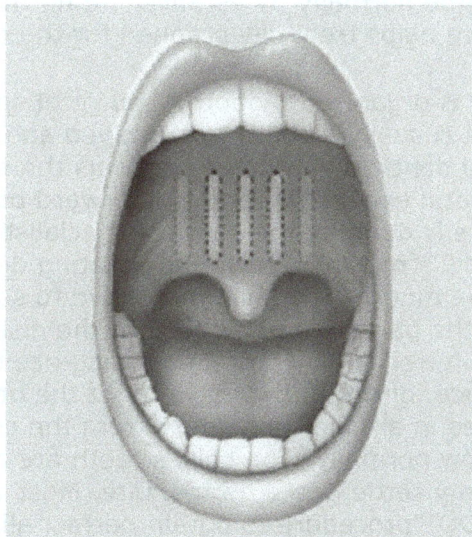

Figure 9.4 The pillar procedure.

AFTER THE SURGERY: You should be able to resume normal activities and eat normally that same day or a day after. Your doctor may prescribe an anti-inflammatory pain medication to keep down swelling and help with any pain you feel after the anesthetic wears off. The patient may also use an antiseptic rinse (mouthwash) for several days and take an antibiotic prescription to prevent future infection.

(iv) IMDO™ for Small Lower Jaw Surgery [13]
MANDIBLE SURGERY

IMDO = Intermolar Mandibular Distraction Osteogenesis

IMDO™ is a unique surgical procedure designed specifically to treat adolescents with a small lower jaw. IMDO™ describes not just the surgical process, but also the wider philosophies for ideal treatment of the small lower jaw.

For those who were born with a small lower jaw, the upper jaw and the nasal airway are often narrow, and there is usually an obstruction of the major airway behind the tongue. This causes snoring and problems with breathing and sleeping, and may even increase the chances of developing sleep apnea in the future. A small lower jaw has speech difficulties, inability to chew normally, and poor jaw or neck posture. It may also cause behavioral changes, poor concentration, and daytime sleepiness, indicating sleep apnea symptoms.

The IMDO™ surgery is mostly performed on children in order to grow or lengthen their lower jaw in all three dimensions to a correct size and proportion so that the lower jaw looks normal.

As the new bone grows between the molars, more room is created to help decrowd the lower teeth. After the surgery, the wisdom teeth may grow and erupt normally, allowing children to keep all of their teeth.

The IMDO™ surgery also brings the main muscles of the tongue forward. This procedure eventually opens, or rather "tents" the major airway behind the tongue. After the surgery, the child would be able to breathe normally by establishing normal SpO2 levels. This obviously means, this procedure helps treat sleep apnea for the children.

THE SURGERY: The IMDO™ is organized by both, a surgical specialist and an orthodontic practitioner. At first the patient (usually a child) is examined and clinical photographs and x-rays are taken. The orthodontic practitioner performs the surgical procedures on the widening of the upper jaw (palatal expansion) and the forward positioning of the upper front teeth. The active-IMDO™ phase is done by the surgical specialist who creates a small separation between the 1st and 2nd molars. Growth stimulating devices called coceancig distractors are placed inside the mouth. The child may have to stay in the hospital for a few days. The doctors would train the parents on how to turn the distractors when at home. Two turns a day per side grows the lower jaw by 1mm, so a distance of 12mm will take about 12 days. The distractors are in place for around 40 days to let the new bone solidify. Everything will then be removed in a minor procedure from the child's mouth, allowing the jaw and face to continue to grow normally. The child's teeth are allowed to naturally decrowd and align, and gradually settle into a normal bite. Most children need orthodontics for a short period after the IMDO™procedure to obtain perfect alignment of their teeth.

Though IMDO™ was designed to treat adolescents in their early to middle teenage years, the procedure has been successfully used in adult patients as well.

The IMDO™ surgery can improve airway volume in the throat, bite relationship, tongue position, jaw posture and neck posture. This improvement would contribute largely to allow more air into the lungs by opening the airway in the throat.

(v) Hyoid Advancement Surgery [14]

The hyoid bone is a small bone in the center of the neck where the muscles of the tongue base and pharynx are joined. Obstructive sleep apnea patients usually have a large tongue, and when they fall asleep, the soft muscles at the base of the tongue are easily relaxed and block the pharynx/windpipe in the throat. The obstruction in the airway of the throat causes obstructive sleep apnea.

In the Hyoid Advancement Surgery, a specially trained surgeon repositions the hypoid bone by placing a suture around it and by suspending it to the front of the lower jaw bone. This minimally-invasive procedure results in expansion of the airway in the throat and prevents the soft tissue from collapsing and blocking the airway when the patient falls asleep. This procedure is usually performed with two small incisions in the neck and is completed in less than one hour. Patients could go home immediately after the surgery and pain is minimal.

Success from this procedure has been outstanding and is becoming a valuable tool in the surgeon's armamentarium.

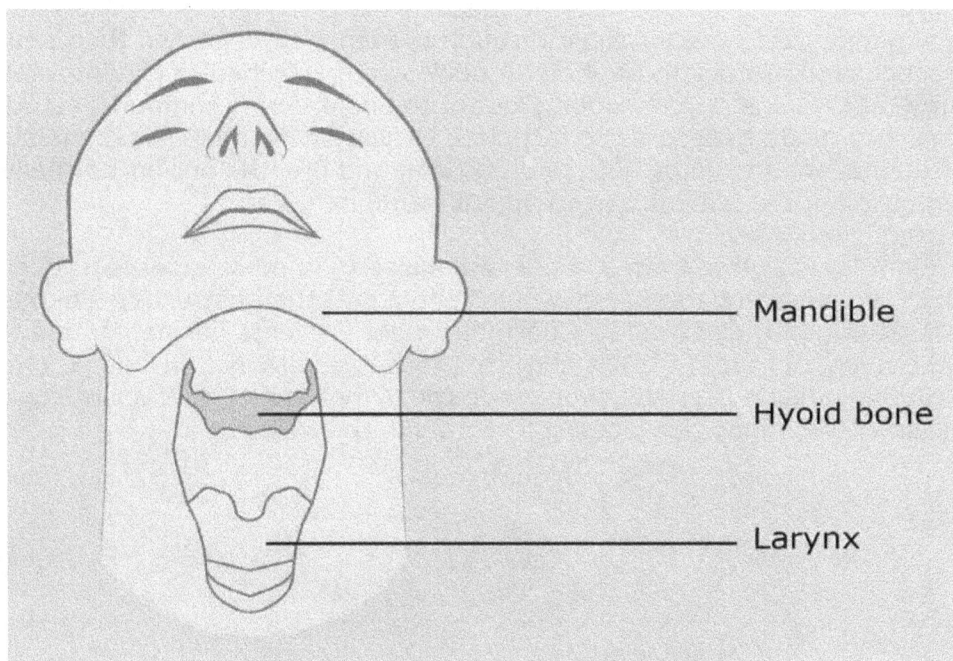

Figure 9.5 Hyoid Advancement Surgery.

(vi) Tongue Advancement Surgery [15]

The largest muscle in the tongue, that runs from the back of the chin (genial tubercles) to the tongue is called the genioglossus. The relaxation of this genioglossus muscle blocks the airway in the throat, causing obstructive sleep apnea. During the surgery, a rectangular cut is made in the jaw bone where the genioglossus muscle is attached. A small titanium plate is used to fix the bone strength to prevent retraction back into the bottom of the mouth. This procedure requires a hospital stay for 1 or 2 days.

(vii) Surgical Tracheostomy [16, 17]

An emergency tracheotomy is performed when your airway gets blocked suddenly, immediately after a traumatic injury to your face or neck. A tracheostomy is also performed when health problems require long-term use of a machine (ventilator) to help you breathe.

Surgical Tracheostomy is performed in a hospital room by a specially trained surgeon. During the procedure, the surgeon makes a horizontal incision through the skin in the lower, front part of the neck. The surgeon pulls the muscles and cuts a small portion of the thyroid gland if needed, and finds the windpipe (trachea) of the airway in the throat. At a specific spot on the windpipe, the surgeon drills a hole and inserts a tracheostomy tube into the hole. A neck strap, attached to the faceplate of the tracheostomy tube, keeps it from slipping out of the hole. Some temporary sutures (stitches) are also made to secure the faceplate to skin of the neck. After the surgery is completed, the patient should be able to breathe in and breathe out air normally. If the surgery is successful, the patient's sleep apnea would be cured.

Minimally-Invasive Tracheostomy is performed in a hospital room by a specially-trained surgeon. During the procedure, the surgeon makes a horizontal incision through the skin in the lower, front part of the neck. A specially designed lens is inserted into the mouth so that the windpipe (trachea) is visible through the lens. The surgeon then drills a hole and inserts a tracheostomy tube into the hole. A neck strap, attached to the faceplate of the tracheostomy tube, keeps it from slipping out of the hole. Some temporary sutures (stitches) are also made to secure the faceplate to skin of the neck. After the surgery is completed, the patient should be able to breathe in and breathe out air normally. If the surgery is successful, the patient's sleep apnea would be cured.

After the patient is recovered from a successful surgery, in most cases, an "overnight pulse oximetry test" or "ploysmnogram test" would reveal that the obstructive sleep apnea is reversed. Desaturation Index would be normal (under 5 events per hour), and the Mean SpO2 would be normal (over 95%). A surgical procedure may not always be one 100% successful. Some patients may still experience the symptoms of mild obstructive sleep apnea because of the minor blockages still remain in the throat.

(viii) Inspire Implant Therapy for Sleep Apnea [18, 19, 20, 21, 22]

Please visit the Inspiresleep website.
https://www.inspiresleep.com/
https://www.inspiresleep.com/faq/

Inspire developed the world's first fully implanted neurostimulation device approved by the United States FDA for the treatment of obstructive sleep apnea (OSA). The Inspire system uses neurostimulation technologies and incorporates a proprietary algorithm that stimulates key airway muscles based on a patient's unique breathing patterns.

Inspire therapy, for obstructive sleep apnea, is an implanted system that senses breathing patterns and delivers mild stimulation to key airway muscles, which keeps the airway open during the sleep. Inspire therapy is designed to reduce the severity of the number of apneas during sleep and improve quality of life for patients who tried the CPAP therapy, could not tolerate the use of the CPAP therapy, and were unable to treat the challenging condition of obstructive sleep apnea.

Inspire Medical Systems, based in Minneapolis, Minnesota, USA, has developed the world's first fully-implanted and FDA-approved neurostimulation system for the treatment of obstructive sleep apnea (OSA). Inspire therapy is controlled with a small, handheld remote, and there is no mask or hose needed. Simply turn the therapy on before you go to bed and off when you wake up. Inspire therapy helps you take control of your sleep apnea and can give you the restful night's sleep you've been missing.

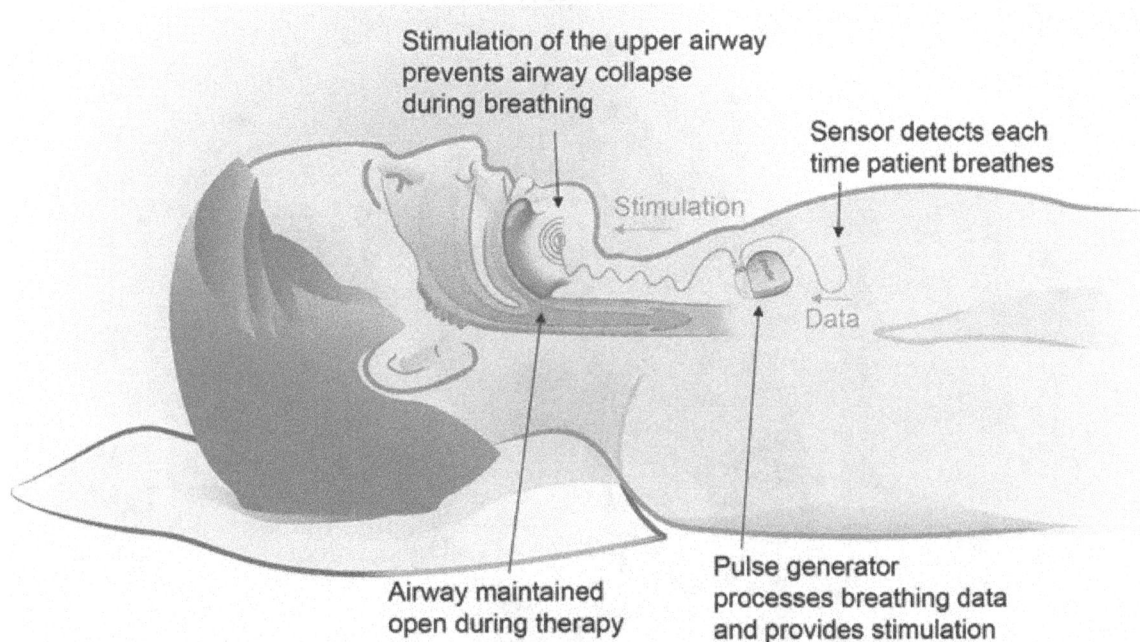

Stimulation of the upper airway prevents airway collapse during breathing

Sensor detects each time patient breathes

Stimulation

Data

Airway maintained open during therapy

Pulse generator processes breathing data and provides stimulation

Courtesy of MetroHealth.org [22]

Figure 9.6 Inspire Implantation Surgery (Upper Airway Stimulation).

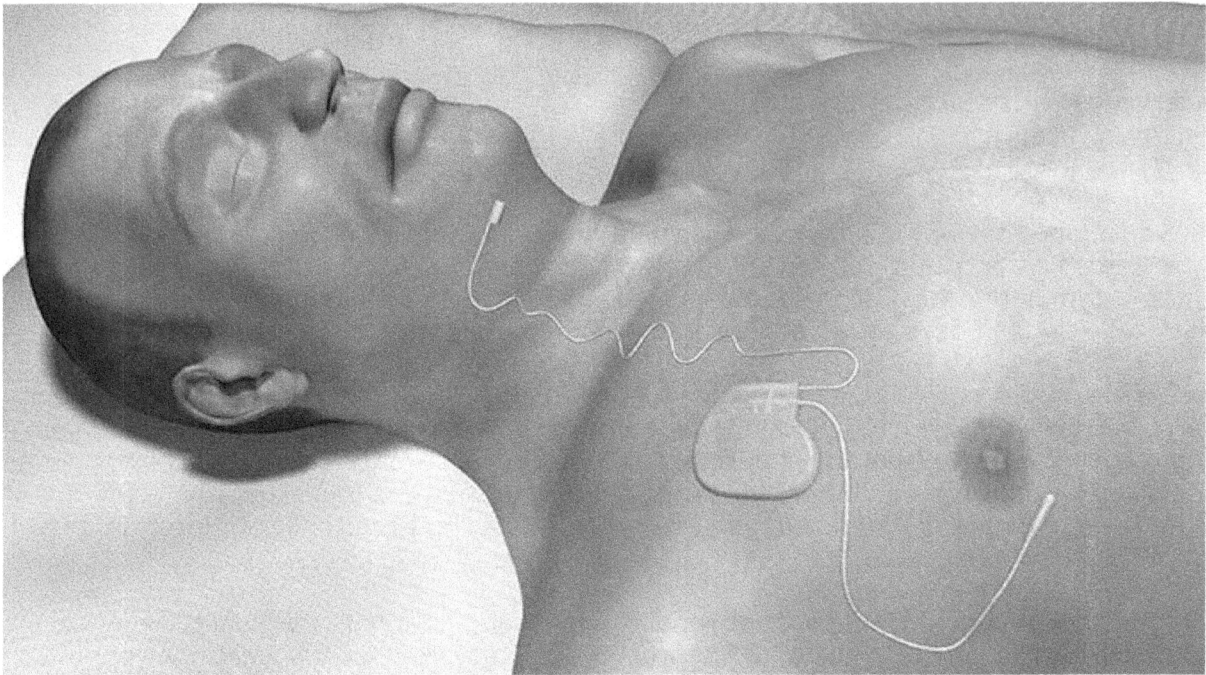

Figure 9.7 Inspire Implantation Surgery (Upper Airway Stimulation).

Inspire works inside your body while you sleep. It's a small device placed during a same-day, outpatient procedure. When you're ready for bed, simply click the remote to turn Inspire on. While you sleep, Inspire opens your airway, allowing you to breathe normally and sleep peacefully. [18, 19, 20, 21, 22, 23, 24, 25]

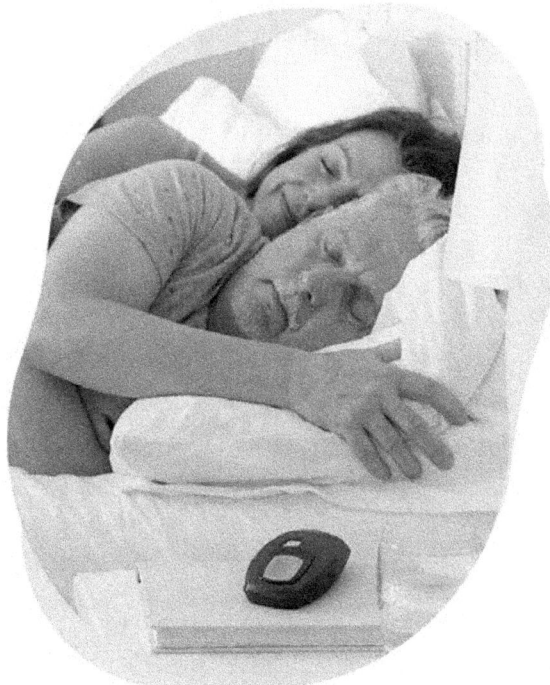

Courtesy of InspireSleep
Figure 9.8 Simply click the remote to turn Inspire on and to keep your airway open.

HOW TO KNOW IF A SURGICAL PROCEDURE IS WORKING OR NOT?
How To Know if Your Sleep Apnea Is Improved or Worsened?

ANSWER: Take the "overnight pulse oximetry test" before and after the surgery, and compare the results (Oxygen Desaturation Index and mean SpO2).

(i) Purchase and learn how to use the Philips Respironics Pulse Oximeter, or Nonin Pulse Oximeter, ResMed Oximeter, Wrist Pulse Oximeter, or any other pulse oximeter to do "overnight pulse oximetry test." Do not rely on cheap devices (they could generate misleading results, so test the device before using it).

(ii) A surgical procedure helps reduce the severity of the sleep apnea disease when a patient has been suffering from severe sleep apnea symptoms, risk factors, side effects and complications. A surgery will definitely and significantly reduce the obstruction in the throat, mouth and nose, and the number desaturation events would significantly be lowered, relieving the pain and discomfort associated with the sleep apnea symptoms.

(iii) After the surgical procedure, and after the patient is recovered from the surgery, take the "overnight pulse oximetry test." If the Desaturation Index is under 5 events per hour and Mean SpO2 (%) is greater than 95%, that means the surgery is one 100% successful.

(iv) However surgery may not be one 100% successful in all cases and for all people. A lot of people after the surgical procedure still live with mild sleep apnea (Desaturation Index would be over 5 events per hour) or moderate sleep apnea (Desaturation Index would be over 15 events per hour). Surgery in many cases helps reduce the severe sleep apnea to moderate or mild sleep apnea. A patient must still treat his/her mild or moderate sleep apnea either by the CPAP therapy, by an oral appliance, or by other therapy.

CHAPTER 9 SLEEP APNEA TREATMENT Section-VII
SURGICAL PROCEDURES

REFERENCES
Obstructive Sleep Apnea in Children

1. Obstructive Sleep Apnea in Children, Authors: James Chan, M.D. Cleveland Clinic Foundation, Cleveland, Ohio, Jennifer C. Edman, M.D., Fairview Hospital, Cleveland, Ohio, Peter J. Koltai, M.D., Cleveland Clinic Foundation, Cleveland, Ohio, American Family Physician, 2004 Mar 1;69(5):1147-1155.
https://www.aafp.org/afp/2004/0301/p1147.html

2. Children's Sleep Apnea by American Sleep Apnea association, 2021.
https://www.sleepapnea.org/treat/childrens-sleep-apnea/

3. Pediatric obstructive sleep apnea by Mayo Clinic, 2021.
https://www.mayoclinic.org/diseases-conditions/pediatric-sleep-apnea/symptoms-causes/syc-20376196

4. Children and Sleep Apnea: What it is, how it harms chilrdrens' sleep and health, and how it can be treated by Sleep Foundation, Updated June 24, 2021.
https://www.sleepfoundation.org/sleep-apnea/children-and-sleep-apnea

5. Obstructive Sleep Apnea in Children by Cedars Sinai, 2021.
https://www.cedars-sinai.org/health-library/diseases-and-conditions---pediatrics/o/obstructive-sleep-apnea-in-children.html

TONSILS AND ADENOIDS

6. Tonsils and Adenoids by Magrabi Hospitals and Centers, Magrabi Hospitals and Centers, Posted on Aug 15, 2015.
https://www.magrabi.com.sa/2015/3552/tonsils-and-adenoids-2/

7. Tonsillectomy and Adenoidectomy for Obstructive Sleep Apnea and Snoring by Healthlink BC, July 24, 2020.
https://www.healthlinkbc.ca/health-topics/hw48845

8. UPPP (Uvulopalatopharyngoplasty) for Obstructive Sleep Apnea by WebMD.
http://www.webmd.com/sleep-disorders/sleep-apnea/uvulopalatopharyngoplasty-for-obstructive-sleep-apnea

9. UPPP (Uvulopalatopharyngoplasty) for Obstructive Sleep Apnea by Calsleep.
http://calsleep.com/services-uppp-california-sleep-doctors-bay-area.html

10. YouTuve Video: Uvulopalatopharyngoplasty (UPPP)- Lateral Expansion Pharyngoplasty Variant with Uvulopalatal Flap, May 27, 2020.
https://www.youtube.com/watch?v=D_UNuOdFbMA

11. Pillar Procedure by Sleep Doctor, 2021.
https://sleep-doctor.com/surgical-treatment-overview/palate-procedures/pillar-procedure/

12. Pillar Procedure by Mayo Clinic, 2021.
https://www.mayoclinic.org/tests-procedures/pillar-procedure/about/pac-20390548

13. IMDO™ is a whole new way to treat a small lower jaw and big overbite by Profilo Surgical Pty Ltd., 2021.
https://profilosurgical.com.au/procedures/imdo

14. HYOID SUSPENSION SURGERY & SLEEP APNEA by NYC Sleep Well, 1175 Park Avenue, Suite 1B, New York, NY 10128.
https://www.nycsleepwell.com/treatment/sleep-apnea-surgical-treatment/hyoid-suspension/

15. Tongue Advancement Surgery, Sleep-apnea-guide.com.
http://www.sleep-apnea-guide.com/genioglossus.html

16. Surgical Tracheostomy by Mayo Clinic, 2021.
http://www.mayoclinic.org/tests-procedures/tracheostomy/details/what-you-can-expect/rec-20234018

17. Surgical Tracheostomy by Mayo Clinic, 2021.
http://www.mayoclinic.org/tests-procedures/tracheostomy/home/ovc-20233993

INSPIRE IMPLANT THERAPY

18. Inspire Upper Airway Stimulator (for Sleep Apnea).
https://www.inspiresleep.com/

19. Frequently Asked Questions, Inspire Upper Airway Stimulator (for Sleep Apnea).
https://www.inspiresleep.com/faq/

20. FDA Approves Inspire® Upper Airway Stimulation (UAS) Therapy for Obstructive Sleep Apnea; Fully Implanted Device Represents New Treatment Option for Patients Unable to Use CPAP.
https://www.inspiresleep.com/press-releases/fda-approves-inspire-upper-airway-stimulation-uas-therapy-for-obstructive-sleep-apnea/

21. Which Patients Are Good Candidates for Inspire Upper Airway Stimulation? Published on February 16, 2016.
http://www.sleepreviewmag.com/2016/02/patients-good-candidates-inspire-upper-airway-stimulation/

22. Inspire Surgery (Upper Airway Stimulation) by MetroHealth,The MetroHealth System, 2500 MetroHealth Drive, Cleveland, OH 44109, Ph: 216-778-7800.
https://www.metrohealth.org/otolaryngology/sleep-surgery/services-we-provide/inspire-surgery

23. What is Hypoglossal Nerve Stimulation Therapy for Sleep Apnea? by Julia Rodriguez, Advanced Sleep Medicine Services, Inc., 2021.
https://www.sleepdr.com/the-sleep-blog/what-is-hypoglossal-nerve-stimulation-therapy-for-sleep-apnea/

24. Don't Like CPAP? An Implantable Device Is Another Option for Your Sleep Apnea, FDA-approved nerve stimulator helps open your airway, by Cleveland Clinic, Posted on January 23, 2019.
https://health.clevelandclinic.org/dont-like-cpap-an-implantable-device-is-another-option-for-your-sleep-apnea/

25. Inspire Hypoglossal Nerve Stimulator Surgery for Sleep Apnea Treatment by Brandon Peters, MD, Verywell Health, Medically reviewed by Kashif J. Piracha, MD, Posted on May 07, 2020.
https://www.verywellhealth.com/inspire-for-sleep-apnea-3015288

CHAPTER 10 SLEEP APNEA TREATMENT Section-VIII
WEIGHT LOSS REVERSES OBSTRUCTIVE SLEEP APNEA
[SCIENTIFIC PROOF EXISTS]

TABLE OF CONTENTS

CHAPTER 10 SCIENTIFIC PROOF EXISTS
WEIGHT LOSS REVERSES OBSTRUCTIVE SLEEP APNEA

All the aforementioned therapies control obstructive sleep apnea, and keep the SpO2 levels normal, only during the usage of the treatment. For example the CPAP keeps the Desaturation Index (number of events/hr) and the SpO2 levels normal only during its usage (during the time when the patient is wearing the device). It is exactly like using eyeglasses for reading. You would be able to see clearly and read when you wear the eyeglasses. But you would not be able to see and read clearly when you don't wear them. The eyeglasses do not cure your eyesight but help control your sight only when you wear them. The CPAP works exactly like that. The CPAP does not cure or reverse sleep apnea but helps you live better during the time you use it.

BUT RESEARCH HAS PROVED WITH SEVERAL REAL-LIFE CASES AND RANDOMIZED STUDIES THAT WEIGHT LOSS CURES AND REVERSES OBSTRUCTIVE SLEEP APNEA.

STUDY PUBLISHED BY Dr. GARY D. FOSTER, PhD, USA [1, 2, 3, 4, 5]

Dr. Gary D. Foster, Ph.D., is Adjunct Professor of Psychology in Psychiatry at the Perelman School of Medicine, University of Pennsylvania. He currently is the Chief Scientific Officer at Weight Watchers International, Inc. Dr. Foster, a clinical psychologist and obesity investigator, was previously the Founder and Director of the Center for Obesity Research and Education at Temple University in Philadelphia, where he was the Laura Carnell Professor of Medicine, Public Health and Psychology.

In 2009 and 2010, Dr. Gary D. Foster and his fellow-researchers published several scientific research papers (the most important one was in the journal "Archives of Internal Medicine") confirming that the symptoms of obstructive sleep apnea and the Desaturation Index (number of sleep apnea events or oxygen desaturation events per hour) can be significantly reduced among obese people by losing at least 10% of the body weight.

The scientific research paper was entitled "A Randomized Study on the Effect of Weight Loss on obstructive sleep apnea Among Obese Patients With Type 2 Diabetes," and the study investigated the effect of weight loss on obstructive sleep apnea in 264 obese adults who were previously diagnosed with obstructive sleep apnea and also with type-2 diabetes. The average weight of the people in the study was 224 pounds. They randomly divided the participants into two groups. The first group participated in the weight loss program with portion-controlled diet and exercise. The second group did not participate in the weight loss program, but received diabetes-management assistance. After one year, the participants in the first group lost an average weight of 24 pounds. But the second group maintained almost the same weight. The research showed that there was a significant reduction of sleep apnea symptoms and severity of sleep apnea among the participants of the first group who lost 24 pounds. Their average Desaturation Index was reduced from 23 events/hr to 13 events/hr. That means that their sleep disorder switched from moderate sleep apnea to mild sleep apnea, which is a significant accomplishment towards curing obstructive sleep apnea. At the same time, the sleep apnea symptoms worsened among the participants of the second group who did not lose weight.

STUDY PUBLISHED BY KAROLINSKA INSTITUTE, SWEDEN [6, 7, 8]

Scientists Dr. Erik Hemmingsson and Dr. Kari Johansson along with their other fellow-researchers published a paper in Dec 2009 in the British Medical Journal, concluding that weight loss can definitely help cure moderate and severe sleep apnea.

The study included 63 obese men (BMI between 30 and 40) aged between 30 and 65. The participants had moderate to severe sleep apnea as measured by the AHI (apnea-hypopnea index). All participants had been on CPAP therapy (a symptom alleviation treatment, which pumps air at a very low pressure and produces more normal breathing patterns through a mask during sleep). The participants were randomly assigned to two groups. The participants of the first group underwent an intense weight-loss program, and the second group served as a control group, for a period of nine weeks.

The results of the study showed that when the participants of the first group lost an average of 19 Kg after nine weeks, their AHI (apnea-hypopnea index) was cut in half or more than half. The researchers very eagerly noticed that the effect of the weight loss program was the greatest in patients with severe sleep apnea. The number of sleep apnea events reduced by more than 58%, indicating that a sleep apnea cure is possible. The patients with the most severe sleep apnea saw the biggest improvements in symptoms and those who lost the most weight improved the most. That means the more severe the sleep apnea symptoms are, the better the effect of the weight loss program on the patients is. They also found that there was no improvement of the sleep apnea symptoms among the participants of the second group who did not undergo the weight-loss program.

To achieve significant weight loss, the participants of the first group were put on a VLCD (Very Low Calorie Diet), which gave them an initial energy input of 554 kcal per day for seven weeks, followed by 1,500 kcal per day for a fortnight during week nine. The control group maintained their normal dietary habits during the nine-week study period, but were afterwards introduced to the VLCD program.

After the VLCD (Very Low Calorie Diet) period, the participants were also invited to take part in a year's behavioral change program to help them maintain their weight loss.

"We often use VLCD in the form of a low calorie powder as part of the treatment of obese patients with a serious comorbidity such as sleep apnea," says Dr. Johansson. "The powder is mixed with water and replaced every meal of the day, which gave a rapid loss of weight. It is also a good way of boosting the patients' motivation."

The researchers stress that the VLCD diet is not a general solution to weight problems, but something mainly to be used in the first phase of a long-term treatment program. To keep the weight off, patients need to work hard to improve their dietary and exercise habits, usually with the aid of a long-term behavior modification program. Drugs can also be used in the post-weight loss phase to further improve weight loss maintenance.

The current study was part funded by Cambridge Manufacturing Company Limited, which markets the Cambridge Diet, the low-calorie powder used in the study. The company had no influence on the study, the analyses or the collation of results. Examples of similar VLCD products marketed by other companies are Nutrilett, Naturdiet and Allevo. The researchers who conducted the study work at the Obesity Unit, Karolinska University Hospital, Huddinge, and the Clinical Epidemiology Unit, Karolinska Institutet, Solna, Stockholm, Sweden.

HOW Dr. RK REVERSED HIS OBSTRUCTIVE SLEEP APNEA?

Introductory Comments

During 2011-2012, I did extensive research on the internet staying up late in the night to find solutions to my medical problems - severe neck pain or stiff neck, lower leg pain or claudication, plantar fasciitis, and others, all of which have been bothering me a lot, for a long time. This kind careless and reckless activity had shifted the biological clock of my brain and, as a result, I developed the Circadian Rhythm Sleep Disorder. I could not fall asleep until 1 am, 2 am or even 3 am. I was sleeping after 3 am and getting up after 1 pm or 2 pm in the afternoon for the last 2-3 years. When I saw my doctor and several specialists, they only prescribed me sleeping pills without addressing the root cause and any pertinent treatment.

During 2011-2014, my plantar fasciitis prevented me from exercising on the treadmill. As a result, I gained some 18 Kg (40 pounds) of body weight. In a routine visit, an endocrinologist suspected that I might be living with sleep apnea when I told him that I had been suffering from uncontrollable weight gain and that I was not sleeping well. The endocrinologist asked me eagerly if I snore a lot and when I said "yes", he referred me to a CPAP vendor called " Independent Respiratory Services (IRS)" and ordered an overnight pulse oximeter test. That CPAP vendor (IRS) diagnosed me with moderate sleep apnea (Desaturation Index was 22 events/hr), and advised me to go on CPAP therapy immediately.

Table 10. 1 Overnight pulse oximetry test results, weight & body mass index.

Date	Waist	Weight	Weight	BMI	Assessment
Units	(Inches)	(Kg)	(Pounds)	(Kg/m ^{2})	
Normal Range	< 34"	< 70 Kg	< 156 lb	18.5 to 24.9	
07-Feb-2015	First Diagnosed with Moderate Sleep Apnea				
	Desaturation Index = 22 Events/hr (by IRS)/				
07-Feb-2015	44	86	191	30.5	Obese
BMI = Weight (Kg) / Height (m) ^{2} = 86 / 1.68 ^{2} = 30.5 = Obese					
07-Apr-2015	Desaturation Index = 28 Events/hr (by Mainland Sleep)				
07-Apr-2015	44	86	191	30.5	Obese

After that I started researching about the CPAP therapy and the local CPAP vendors. From my own research, I chose to purchase the CPAP machine and accessories from another CPAP vendor called "Mainland Sleep". I took my "overnight pulse oximetry test" again on April 7, 2015, and I was shocked to learn that my Desturation Index rose to 28 events/hour, which means I was about to be diagnosed with severe sleep apnea. I knew that with severe sleep apnea, I could suffocate myself, and the blocked airway could kill me in my sleep. Many people died like that.
16-Mar-2015 CPAP Therapy started seriously.

I immediately took action. I AWAKENED THE GIANT WITHIN MYSELF. I started researching about this topic more seriously than ever before. My extensive reading and research suggested that I need to lose weight immediately. In March 2015, I purchased a pair of oversized Hoka shoes, and dressed them with 3 layers of soft cushion to protect my feet from plantar fasciitis, and started using the treadmill every day (7 days a week) for 1 to 2 hours. I lost some weight, but it was an uphill battle as I felt that I was fighting against a devil because my weight loss was found to be sluggish no matter how hard I tried. I personally experienced for a long time that sleep apnea prevents weight loss (TRUE!). The rest of the story can be understood by reading through the table shown below.

THE SLEEP APNEA AND WEIGHT-LOSS JOURNAL OF
Dr. RK Using Weight-Loss Diet Level-I (2000 Calories)

Table 10.2 Overnight pulse oximetry test results & weight loss data.

Date	Waist	Weight	Weight	BMI	Assessment
Units	(Inches)	(Kg)	(Pounds)	(Kg/m ^{2})	
Normal Range	< 34"	< 70 Kg	< 156 lb	18.5 to 24.9	
07-Feb-2015	First Diagnosed with Moderate Sleep Apnea (Index=22 to 28 Events/hr)				
07-Feb-2015	44	86	191	30.5	Obese
BMI = Weight (Kg) / Height (m) ^{2} = 86 / 1.68 ^{2} = 30.5 = Obese					
19-Feb-2015	Committed to Lose Weight; Started Weight-Loss Diet (Level-I)				
12-Mar-2015	Started Exercising Every Day in the Gym (60 to 80 minutes/day).				
17-Apr-2015	43	84	187	29.8	Overweight
01-May-2015	42	83	184	29.4	Overweight
23-May-2015	42	84	187	29.8	Overweight
03-Jul-2015	41	82	182	29.1	Overweight
11-Jul-2015	40	80.5	179	28.5	Overweight
31-Jul-2015	39	80	178	28.3	Overweight
03-Aug-2015	39	79	176	28.0	Overweight
20-Aug-2015	39	80	178	28.3	Overweight
31-Aug-2015	39	80	178	28.3	Overweight
In 7 months, I lost only 6 Kg (13 Pounds); My weight loss was slow!					
My weight reached plateau; My sleep apnea is preventing my weight loss.					
08-Sep-2015	39	79	176	28.0	Overweight
06-Oct-2015	38	78.5	174	27.8	Overweight
11-Oct-2015	38	78.5	174	27.8	Overweight
10-Nov-2015	38	78.5	174	27.8	Overweight
25-Dec-2015	37	78	173	27.6	Overweight
28-Dec-2015	Oximetry Test Done: Desaturation Index = 6.9-8.4 Events/hr				
	I still have mild sleep apnea; However my weight reached plateau!				
14-Jan-2016	36.5	77	171	27.3	Overweight
19-Mar-2016	36	76.5	170	27.1	Overweight
19-Mar-2016	Oximetry Test Done: Desaturation Index = 4.6-4.8 Events/hr				
	I still have mild sleep apnea; However my weight reached plateau!				
27-May-2016	37	78	173	27.6	Overweight
12-Sep-2016	38.5	78	173	27.6	Overweight
My Weight Loss Was Very Slow; My Belly Fat and Weight Started Going Up.					
I Took Action; I Decided to Do Something About It and Researched.					
I Created Weight-Loss Diet (Level-II), Which Helped Me Loss Weight Fast.					

Table 10.3 Assessment guidelines for sleep apnea and weight loss.

Desaturation Index	Assessment		BMI (Kg/m^2)	Assessment
0 - 4 Events/hr	Normal (No Sleep Apnea)		< 18.5	Underweight
5 - 14 Events/hr	Mild Sleep Apnea		18.5 to 24.9	Normal
15 - 29 Events/hr	Moderate Sleep Apnea		25.0 to 29.9	Overweight
≥ 30 Events/hr	Severe Sleep Apnea		≥ 30	Obese

DISCUSSION OF TABLE 10.2: As shown in Table 10.2, when I was first diagnosed with obstructive sleep apnea, my "overnight pulse oximetry test" done on 07-Feb-2015 showed that my Desaturation Index was 22 events/hr. When I repeated the test on 07-Apr-2015, my desaturation index went up to 28 events/hr, which means my sleep disorder was almost approaching severe sleep apnea (if the Desaturation Index is ≥ 30 events/hr, that indicates severe sleep apnea). My extensive reading and research suggested me that I need to lose weight immediately. So I started losing weight by using the weight-loss diet (level-I).

As shown in Table 10.2, when I tried the weight-loss diet (level-I) for 20 months, my weight dropped from 86 Kg (190 lb) to 78 Kg (175 lb). I lost only 8 Kg or 18 pounds. I needed to lose at least another 8 Kg or 18 pounds to attain normal body weight. I checked everything, and found the following flaws.

I Found the Following Flaws While On The Weight-Loss Diet (Level-I):
1. MAJOR OBSTACLE: MY SLEEP APNEA HAD BEEN PREVENTING MY WEIGHT LOSS.
• The stress that sleep apnea causes on heart and brain of a person can be so severe and harmful that long-term health consequences could include cognitive deficits.
• Cognitive deficits, also known as intellectual disability, occurs when problems with thought processes occur due to lack of sufficient oxygen supply to the brain. It can include a temporary or permanent loss of mental functions, loss of higher reasoning, forgetfulness, learning disabilities, and other weird behavior.
• When someone has sleep apnea, their brain mistakenly thinks that they would be starving in the near future, and causes the liver to store and hold the fat for the future use.
2. Also when I had sleep apnea, my SpO2 levels (percentage saturation of oxygen in the blood) used to drop significantly and would not be normal throughout the night. So my resting metabolism slowed down, resulting in sluggish weight loss or no weight loss.
3. My metabolism most probably slowed down because of my age (I was getting older) after I was diagnosed with obstructive sleep apnea, keeping my weight constant no matter how hard I tried to lose it.
4. My lower leg pain and my plantar fasciitis did not allow me to do high-intensity exercise so I was not burning sufficient calories during exercise. As a result, the stubborn fat in my belly refused to melt away for a long time.
5. I did not exercise high willpower and high self-discipline right from the beginning. I had been cheating on my diet, and was consuming junk foods in restaurants.

JUNK FOODS are strategically manufactured from both processed foods and refined foods, adding large quantities of sugar, salt, oil, fat and several other chemicals including artificial colors and flavors to boost our cravings. This makes us buy more and eat more. Junk foods sabotage our weight-loss efforts. I had been eating junk foods here and there, consuming pizza slices, chicken donair in middle eastern places, pita bread, whole wheat bread, deep-fried samosas and spring rolls, Oh HENRY bars, chocolate chewy candies, dipped cone ice creams, cashew clusters, Diet Cokes, Diet Pepsis, excessive fruits and plenty of other snacks every now and then, which was certainly a major mistake.

<u>So I decided to put an end to consuming junk foods by exercising high willpower and high self-discipline</u>. Healthy eating habits are essential to practice any weight-loss plan. This decision has helped me tremendously to quick-start my own weight-loss plan. The fat in my belly melted away quickly and easily day by day when I started my weight-loss diet (level-II).

I Took Action and Created the Weight-Loss Diet (Level-II)

1. I drastically reduced the daily calorie instate from 2000 Kcal to 1000 Kcal. I started eating whole foods only, and eliminated all junk foods made from processed and refined foods from my meal plan.

2. I drastically reduced the fat content (to almost zero) in my diet. Because I did not consume fat, my body ate my own fat, which helped me lose weight rapidly.

3. I eliminated all animal products (chicken and fish that I was eating before) from my diet as they contain high fat.

4. I exercised high willpower and high self-discipline. I wanted to lose weight and reverse my sleep apnea. I stopped eating all junk foods made from processed and refined foods and started eating whole foods strictly.

5. I minimized my salt and oil consumption. (I was consuming too much salt and oil before.)

6. I replaced all my in-between meal snacks with the crunchy and tasty organic Kamut Puffs.

7. I introduced organic apple cider vinegar with the mother, unpasteurized and unfiltered into my diet. I started taking it 2 to 3 times a day using a straw, which probably contributed to some extent in my weight loss program.

8. I started drinking 16 cups of purified water per day as compared to 8 cups per day.

9. I did not have hunger attacks, and had no cravings of any kind even though I drastically reduced my daily calorie intake and consumed only 1000 Kcal per day. My energy levels were normal.

10. It is important to note here that I never took any hunger suppressants prescribed by any doctor. All my weight-loss attempts were one 100% natural.

11. When I created the Weight-Loss Diet (Level-II) and stopped eating all junk foods made from processed and refined foods, and started eating only whole foods, the fat in my belly melted away day by day, right in front of my eyes. Beating all odds, I lost weight and my body attained normal weight within 6 weeks. My Body Mass Index (BMI) reached perfectly normal. More interestingly, my obstructive sleep apnea (OSA) disappeared. My Oxygen Desaturation Index (ODI) decreased from a high risk 28 events/hr to a stunning 0.6 event/hr.

SLEEP APNEA AND WEIGHT-LOSS JOURNAL OF Dr. RK
Using Weight-Loss Diet Level-II (1000 Calories)
HIGH WILLPOWER & HIGH SELF-DESCIPLINE REQUIRED!

I had been cheating on my diet, and was consuming junk foods here and there. Then I strictly enforced a LAW on myself not to eat junk foods anymore, but instead eat only home-cooked meals made from whole foods. I carefully eliminated all processed and refined foods from my diet. When I did that, and when I drastically reduced my daily calorie intake from 2000 Kcal to 1000 Kcal, my belly fat melted away day by day, right in front of my eyes. I lost weight and my BMI reached normal as shown in the table below. Following is the Proof That obstructive sleep apnea Can Be Reversed By Losing Weight!

Table 10.4 Overnight pulse oximetry test results & weight loss data.

Date	Waist	Weight	Weight	BMI	Assessment
Units	(Inches)	(Kg)	(Pounds)	(Kg/m ^{2})	
Normal Range	< 34"	< 70 Kg	< 156 lb	18.5 to 24.9	
14-Sep-2016	Started Weight-Loss Diet (Level-II); 1000 Calories/Day.				
	Started Doing Treadmill & Bike Every Day (60 to 90 min per day).				
14-Sep-2016	38.5	78	173	27.6	Overweight
BMI = Weight (Kg) / Height (m) ^{2} = 78 / 1.68 ^{2} = 27.6 = Overweight					
15-Sep-2016	37	77	171	27.3	Overweight
18-Sep-2016	37	76	169	26.9	Overweight
19-Sep-2016	36	75	167	26.6	Overweight
27-Sep-2016	36	74	164	26.2	Overweight
02-Oct-2016	35.5	73.5	163	26.0	Overweight
02-Oct-2016	35.5	73.5	163	26.0	Overweight
02-Oct-2016	35.5	73.5	163	26.0	Overweight
04-Oct-2016	35	73	162	25.9	Overweight
11-Oct-2016	34	72	160	25.5	Overweight
18-Oct-2016	34	71	158	25.2	Overweight
27-Oct-2016	34	70	156	24.8	Normal
09-Nov-2016	33	69	153	24.4	Normal
18-Nov-2015	Oximetry Test Done: Desaturation Index = 1.2-1.3 Events/hr)				
22-Nov-2016	33	68.5	152	24.3	Normal
23-Nov-2016	32.5	68	151	24.1	Normal
29-Nov-2015	Oximetry Test Done: Desaturation Index = 0.6 Events/hr.				
When my body resumed normal weight, my sleep apnea disappeared.					
01-Dec-2016	32.5	68	151	24.1	Normal
08-Dec-2016	32.5	67.5	150	23.9	Normal
01-Jan-2017	33	68	151	24.1	Normal
05-Jan-2017	32	67	149	23.7	Normal
11-Jan-2017	32	67	149	23.7	Normal

THE OVERNIGHT PULSE OXIMETRY TEST RESULTS OF Dr. RK
Overnight Oximetry Tests by Mainland Sleep Diagnostics Ltd., Burnaby, BC, Canada

07-Apr-2015 This Was My SpO2 Chart When I was Diagnosed With Moderate Sleep Apnea.

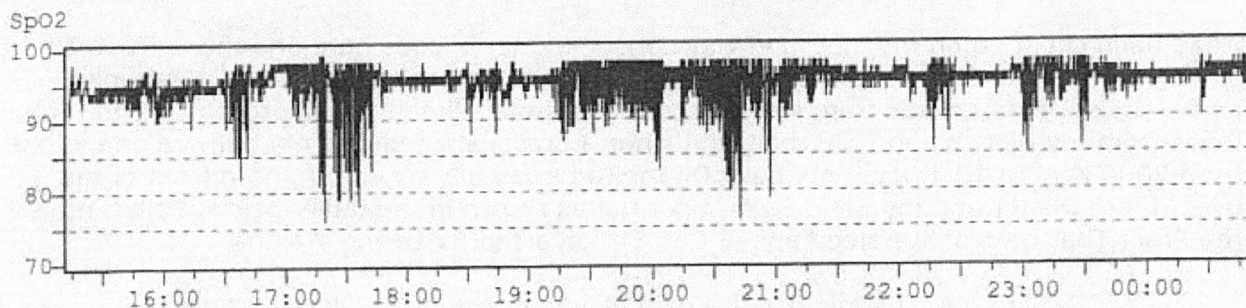

Desaturation Index = 28 Events/hr; Weight = 86 Kg/191 Lbs; BMI = 30.5 (Obese)
Highest SpO2 = 99%; Lowest SpO2 = 76%; Mean SpO2 = 95%

18-Nov-2016 This Was My SpO2 Chart After I Reversed My Sleep Apnea.
Wide Fluctuations of SpO2 Have Been Treated and Minimized.

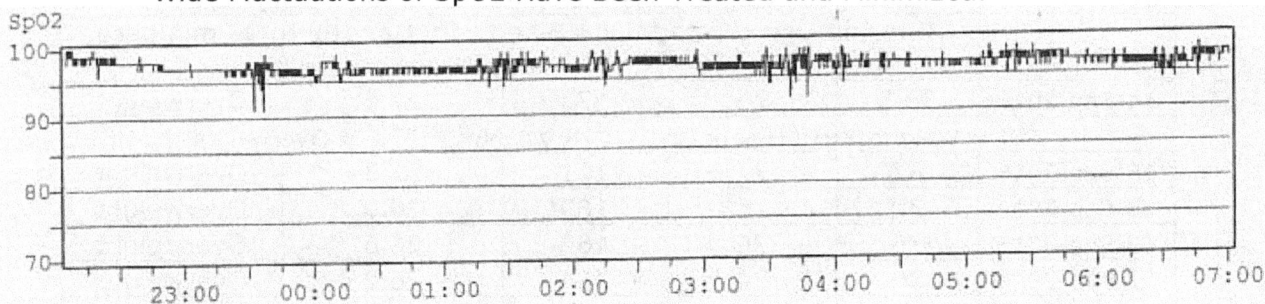

Desaturation Index = 1.2 Events/hr; Weight = 68 Kg/151 Lbs; BMI = 24.1 (Normal)
Highest SpO2 = 99%; Lowest SpO2 = 91%; Mean SpO2 = 97%

20-Nov-2016 This Was My SpO2 Chart When I Used CPAP Recently.
CPAP Pressure = 7 – 11 cm H_2O;   AHI (from CPAP Report) = 1.2 Events/hr

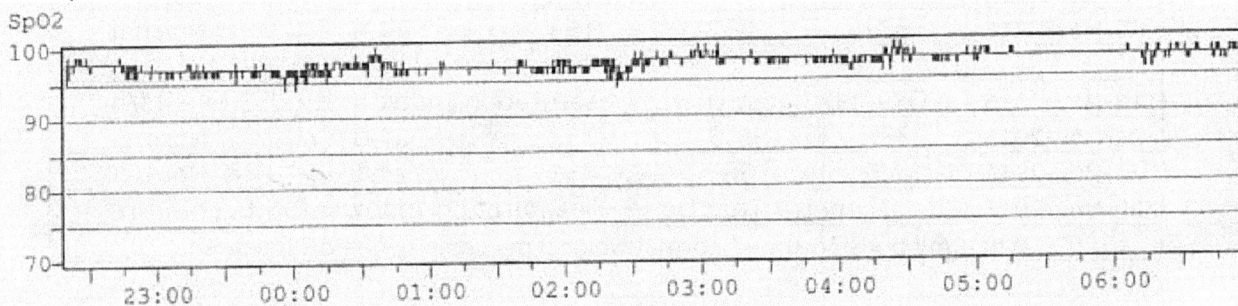

Desaturation Index = 1.0 Events/hr; Weight = 68 Kg/151 Lbs; BMI = 24.1 (Normal)
Highest SpO2 = 100%; Lowest SpO2 = 94%; Mean SpO2 = 97.50%

Figure 10.1 SpO2 versus time chart when diagnosed with sleep apnea and when reversed.

INTERPRETATION OF THE OVERNIGHT PULSE OXIMETRY TEST RESULTS OF Dr. RK

WHEN MY BODY RESUMED NORMAL WEIGHT, MY SLEEP APNEA DISAPPEARED!

SYNOPSIS: As shown in the aforementioned tables (Table 10.2 & Table 10.4), when I was first diagnosed with obstructive sleep apnea, my overnight pulse oximtetry test done on 07-Feb-2015 showed that my Desaturation Index was 22 events/hr. When I repeated the test on 07-Apr-2015, my Desaturation Index went up to 28 events/hr, which means I would soon be diagnosed with severe sleep apnea (if the Desaturation Index is ≥ 30 events/hr, that indicates severe sleep apnea).

With severe sleep apnea, I knew that I could suffocate myself due to the blocked airway and could die in my sleep. It could happen any time if I live with negligence. I therefore took action and awakened the giant within myself. My extensive reading and research suggested me that "I need to lose weight fast." I was then committed to losing weight and created my very own weight-loss diet incorporating daily exercise (running on a treadmill every day). It was like an uphill battle. It was exactly like fighting against a devil because sleep apnea prevents weight loss. Even if I went to gym and ran on a treadmill twice a day, the stubborn fat refused to melt away for a long time.

But my further reading and research suggested me that I needed to do some adjustments to my diet and lower the calories being consumed from junk foods. I learned that when calories being burned by my body are more than the calories being consumed, I would lose weight. I then created a new weight-loss diet, by making drastic changes to my diet by incorporating whole foods only, and by removing all processed foods and refined foods. As a result, my weight started melting away day by day right in front of my eyes, and I accomplished my weight loss goal.

After losing 40 pounds of weight and 12 inches around the waist, naturally without ever using drugs or supplements, my weight dropped from 190 pounds to 150 pounds, my Body Mass Index (BMI) dropped from 30.5 (obese) to 24.1 (perfectly normal). The Oxygen Desaturation Index (ODI) from an "overnight pulse oximetry test" dropped from a high-risk 28 events/hr to a stunning 0.6 event/hr in 22 months, and I completely reversed my obstructive sleep apnea.

The CPAP therapy, being the best treatment available currently, controls sleep apnea and keeps the SpO2 level (percentage saturation of blood oxygen level) and Desaturation Index perfectly normal only during the time you wear the CPAP machine correctly and use it correctly. It is important to note here that CPAP therapy does not heal, cure or reverse sleep apnea. But weight loss gradually heals, cures and reverses obstructive sleep apnea.

However I must watch my weight constantly and prevent it from regaining through caution, care, self-discipline and willpower. As long as I maintain the normal body weight, and maintain normal body mass index (BMI), my obstructive sleep apnea should remain reversed for the rest of my life.

AUTHOR'S UPDATE

During 2015-2016, when I lost 40 pounds of my body weight and when my body resumed perfectly normal weight, I not only reversed my obesity but also simultaneously reversed my obstructive sleep apnea and my chronic insomnia. Immediately after I lost 40 pounds, I have slowly introduced the following changes to my daily diet routine and my lifestyle during the past 5 years (during 2016-2021):

(i) I have slowly introduced oven-baked skinless chicken, turkey or fish into my Egg White Omelet recipe.

(ii) I started eating my breakfast daily: one baked whole wheat pita bread after spreading a tablespoon of creamy organic coconut oil, and a cup of organic coffee.

(iii) I sometimes even replace my Egg-White Omelet with a home-cooked meal made from brown rice, rotisserie chicken (or fish), a variety of organic vegetables, greens, leafy vegetables, chickpeas, kidney beans and organic yogurt.

(iv) I started eating unsalted and dry-roasted cashews, walnuts, soaked almonds, blanched almonds, and protein bars as my in-between meal snacks on an irregular basis. I regularly eat organic Kamut puffs and organic fruits as my in-between meal snack to avoid being hungry.

(v) I sometimes even cheat on my diet, and eat deep-fried French fries, hashbrowns, samosas, spring rolls, and Oh Henry bars (which are my favorite snacks) once or twice a week.

(vi) I even started eating at a buffet (a heavy meal of all kinds of unlimited items of food including the dessert) in restaurants once every week or once every fortnight. Whenever I eat a heavy meal in a restaurant, I do not eat any other meals (except a few fruits) on that day. That means I eat only one meal on that day whenever I eat a heavy meal in a restaurant.

(vii) However I never discontinued or skipped my daily exercise program, not even a day. Every day (7 days a week) I go to gym and do 1 hour of treadmill, or at least 30 minutes of treadmill and 30 minutes of bike or other equipment.

Miraculously, my weight remained steady and normal at 150 pounds during the past 5 years (2016-2021). And I am confident that my weight will remain steady and normal for the rest of my life. I now know how to keep my weight perfectly normal and well controlled.

LEARNED LESSON: As long as my body weight remains perfectly normal, my obstructive sleep apnea would remain reversed.

CHAPTER 10 WEIGHT LOSS REVERSES OBSTRUCTIVE SLEEP APNEA [SCIENTIFIC PROOF EXISTS]

REFERENCES
Weight Loss Indeed Reverses Obstructive Sleep Apnea: There are Scientific Journal Publications

1. 8Obstructive Sleep Apnea and Diabetes: What We Know and What Can Be Done? by Gary D. Foster, Ph.D, Temple University School of Medicine, Monday, June 21, 2010.
http://www.diabetescare.net/article/title/obstructive-sleep-apnea-and-diabetes-what-we-know-and-what-can-be-done

2. JOURNAL REFERENCE & JOURNAL PUBLICATION, Sept 28, 2009.
Arch Intern Med. 2009;169(17):1619-1626. doi:10.1001/archinternmed.2009.266.
A Randomized Study on the Effect of Weight Loss on Obstructive Sleep Apnea Among Obese Patients With Type 2 Diabetes: The Sleep AHEAD Study. Gary D. Foster, PhD; Kelley E. Borradaile, PhD; Mark H. Sanders, MD; et al.
http://jamanetwork.com/journals/jamainternalmedicine/article-abstract/224770

3. Weight Loss Helps Sleep Apnea, Shedding Extra Pounds May Relieve or Even Cure Obstructive Sleep Apnea Symptoms, by Jennifer Warner, Sept. 28, 2009.
http://www.webmd.com/sleep-disorders/sleep-apnea/news/20090928/weight-loss-helps-sleep-apnea

4. Losing Weight to Reverse Sleep Apnea by David Mendosa, Published On: October 11, 2009.
http://www.healthcentral.com/diabetes/c/17/90297/losing-reverse-sleep/

5. Long-Term Effect of Weight Loss on Obstructive Sleep Apnea Severity in Obese Patients with Type 2 Diabetes. Sleep. 2013 May 1; 36(5): 641–649.
Published online 2013 May 1. doi: 10.5665/sleep.2618.
https://www.ncbi.nlm.nih.gov/pmc/articles/PMC3624818/

6. Weight-loss proves an effective cure for sleep apnoea, Karolinska Institutet, Sweden.
Effect of a very low energy diet on moderate and severe obstructive sleep apnoea in obese men: a randomised controlled trial. Publication: Johansson K, Neovius M, Lagerros Y, Harlid R, Rössner S, Granath F, et al, BMJ 2009 Dec;339():b4609. Published 2009-12-04 00:00. Updated 2014-02-21 10:45.
http://ki.se/en/news/weight-loss-proves-effective-cure-for-sleep-apnoea

7. WEIGHT LOSS REVERSES OSA (Obstructive Sleep Apnea), by Science Daily.
Karolinska Institute, A Medical University, Solna, Stockholm, Sweden.
https://www.sciencedaily.com/releases/2009/12/091203222145.htm

8. Weight Loss May Improve Sleep Apnea (Karolinska Institute, A Medical University, Solna, Stockholm, Sweden): Study Shows Weight Loss Has Long-Term Benefits in Treating Sleep Apnea by Salynn Boyles, WebMD.
http://www.webmd.com/sleep-disorders/sleep-apnea/news/20110601/weight-loss-may-improve-sleep-apnea#1

CHAPTER 11 RECOMMENDATIONS ON
REVERSING OBSTRUCTIVE SLEEP APNEA

TABLE OF CONTENTS

CHAPTER 11 RECOMMENDATIONS ON
REVERSING OBSTRUCTIVE SLEEP APNEA

The following recommendations would certainly help you reverse obstructive sleep apnea.

	SHORTLIST OF RECOMMENDATIONS
1	Understand and master the sleep apnea terminology with clear concept.
2	Learn how to purchase & use the pulse oximeter confidently. Do your own overnight pulse oximetry test at home always trying to lower your Desaturation Index & to increase Mean SpO2 Level.
3	Learn how to use the CPAP machine and mask confidently.
4	Learn how to treat wide fluctuations of SpO2 level during the sleep.
5	Learn how to calculate your excess body weight. And learn how to lose all your excess body weight. There is scientific proof that sleep apnea can be reversed by losing weight.
6	Follow all recommendations provided in this chapter carefully.

INTRODUCTION TO REVERSING OBSTRUCTIVE SLEEP APNEA

a. YES, IT IS POSSIBLE TO REVERSE SLEEP APNEA (there are scientific publications) if you are obese or overweight and if you are diagnosed with obstructive sleep apnea due to excess body weight gained over years. You can definitely reverse your obstructive sleep apnea by losing all that excess body weight by exercising high self-discipline and high willpower. But you should make sure that you have lost all that excess body weight by performing the body mass index (BMI) calculation, or by monitoring body fat percentage from a device.

Even if you cannot reverse your sleep apnea completely by losing weight because you are unable to lose all your excess body weight even though you tried hard, you can always attempt to lower your your Desaturation Index (number of sleep apnea events per hour) and increase your Mean SpO2 level by losing at least some of your excess body weight. Whenever your Desaturation Index is lowered and mean SpO2 level is increased, you feel a lot better and your overall health improves.

<u>If your Desaturation Index (events/hr) is under 5, and also if your Mean SpO2 level is over 95% from an "overnight pulse oximetry test," that means your sleep apnea is completely reversed.</u>

b. NO, IT IS NOT POSSIBLE TO REVERSE SLEEP APNEAS if you have chronic nasal congestion, unusual blockages in your mouth, nose and throat, unusual tongue size, enlarged tonsils or adenoids, oversized uvula, oversized tongue, or a small and undersized jaw, and other kinds of blockages in your breathing system located near the airway of your throat.

However you can always attempt to lower your your Desaturation Index (number of sleep apnea events per hour) and increase your Mean SpO2 level by losing your excess body weight if you are overweight or obese under these circumstances. Whenever your Desaturation Index is lowered and Mean SpO2 level is increased, your overall health improves, and you feel a lot better. And all risk factors would be minimized!

I. MASTER THE "TERMINOLOGY" OF THE SLEEP APNEA

(i) SpO2 (Blood Oxygen Saturation, Expressed as a Percentage)
(ii) Mean SpO2, Lowest SpO2 & Highest SpO2
(iii) Oxygen Desaturation Index (ODI) or Desaturation Index (DI)
(iv) Apnea Hypopnea Index (AHI)

Please refer to Chapter 2, read and understand the above-mentioned terms with clear concept.

Table 11.1 Assessment guidelines of sleep apnea using DI and AHI.

Desaturation Index	SpO2 Level	Assessment
0 - 4 Events/hr	96% - 99%	Normal (No Sleep Apnea)
5 - 14 Events/hr	90% - 95%	Mild Sleep Apnea
15 - 29 Events/hr	80% - 90%	Moderate Sleep Apnea
≥ 30 Events/hr	< 80%	Severe Sleep Apnea

AHI	SpO2 Level	Assessment
0 - 4 Events/hr	96% - 99%	Normal (No Sleep Apnea)
5 - 14 Events/hr	90% - 95%	Mild Sleep Apnea
15 - 29 Events/hr	80% - 90%	Moderate Sleep Apnea
≥ 30 Events/hr	< 80%	Severe Sleep Apnea

Normal SpO2 Level
Normal/Healthy oxygen saturation level (SpO2 level), at sea level, **should be between 96% and 99%**.

• You should make sure that your SpO2 level is normal during the day and during the night. During the day, or any time, you can check your SpO2 level by using a Spotcheck Oximeter.

• But if you suffer from sleep apnea, your SpO2 level goes down below normal during the night while sleeping. To find out how low your SpO2 level is going down during the sleep, you should use "Overnight Pulse Oximeter for Continuous Monitoring" by sleeping with Pulse Oximeter in the night. By uploading the data from the Pulse Oximeter to your computer early in the morning, you can find out the Desturation Index (Number of sleep apnea events per hour), Minimum SpO2, Maximum SpO2, and Mean SpO2 level. Please refer to Chapter 2.

a. All the above-mentioned terms are explained in Chapter 2. AHI (Apnea Hypopnea Index) is used in the CPAP report whereas Desaturation Index, Mean SpO2, Lowest SpO2 & Highest SpO2 are used in the "overnight pulse oximetry test results." When you use the CPAP machine, every morning, you should check your CPAP report on on your CPAP machine, and also on your computer, and make sure that the AHI is under 5 events per hour. If AHI is 5 or more than 5 events per hour, that means the CPAP machine is not working or broke down, and/or there could be leaks in your CPAP mask. You should take it back to your doctor or the CPAP vendor where you purchased it, and make sure that the CPAP machine works perfectly. The pressure should be adjusted untik the AHI is under 5.

b. If your AHI from your CPAP report is normal (under 5), it does not mean that your Desaturation Index (number of sleep apnea events per hour) from the "overnight pulse oximetry test" would also be normal (When you take the "overnight pulse oximetry test," you must not wear your CPAP). Your AHI remains normal only during the night you slept with your CPAP machine, and it does not tell anything about your sleep apnea progress or about your sleep disorder. The Desaturation Index (number of sleep apnea events per hour) from an "overnight pulse oximetry test" tells you the whole story about your sleep apnea progress or about your sleep disorder. Once every few months, you should take the "overnight pulse oximetry test" to check your sleep apnea progress.

c. Whenever you take the home-based "overnight pulse oximetry test," you should discontinue your CPAP at least for a week before taking the test. Then only you can confidently confirm that your results obtained from the overnight oximetry test are accurate. Whenever you take the "overnight pulse oximetry test," in the following morning, you should eagerly check your results focussing your attention on Desaturation Index and Mean SpO2. You should eagerly look for these 2 results and check if these results are normal or not. If they are not normal, you should take action and try to lose more excess body weight, and try to further lower your Desaturation index and Mean SpO2. If these two results are normal, that means your sleep apnea is reversed.

d. Find out the severity of your obstructive sleep apnea (mild, moderate or severe) by taking the home-based "overnight pulse oximetry test." Make sure the oximetry test results are reliable. Whenever you do the home-based oximetry test, do it by using two different oximeters (two meters borrowed from two different CPAP vendors, or one meter borrowed from the CPAP vendor, and another meter borrowed from your doctor's sleep clinic) and compare the results. The CPAP vendors sometimes carry and lend you broken oximeters and print wrong results. Therefore you should be extra-cautious, and make sure that the results generated from the "overnight pulse oximetry test" are gnuine and accurate.

e. You could also purchase a pulse oximeter online and do your own oximetry test and compare the results with those obtained from the oximeter you borrowed from the CPAP vendor or from your doctor's sleep clinic. When you purchase it online, the seller is supposed to teach you over the phone on how to use the meter and how to do the "overnight pulse oximetry test." You can learn everything over the phone, and start using your own meter purchased. With a little extra effort, you can master the art of using an oximeter to determine the severity of your obstructive sleep apnea. By knowing the desaturation index (number of oxygen desaturation events per hour) reliably, you would know the severity of your obstructive sleep apnea (mild, moderate or severe).

f. You should do this "overnight pulse oximetry test" on your own without depending on your doctors, CPAP vendors or hospitals if you want reverse or improve your sleep apnea. When you are able to do this test on your own confidently, you can go fast on reversing sleep apnea or at least reduce the severity of the sleep apnea (mild, moderate or severe) and the underlying symptoms.

g. Make sure you understand the results obtained from the "overnight pulse oximetry test" clearly. You should possess an expert knowledge and total command on the aforementioned terminology and tests if you want to reverse or improve your obstructive sleep apnea.

II. LEARN HOW TO PURCHASE & USE THE PULSE OXIMETER FOR CONTINUOUS MONITORING

Purchase one of the following pulse oximeters for Continuous Monitoring:
a. Philips Respironics 920M Handheld Pulse Oximeter [30]
b. Nonin-8500 Handheld Pulse Oximeter [31]
c. Wrist Watch Pulse Oximeter (less expensive unit) [32a, 32b]
   ToronTek-B400 Oximeter or CMS50F Oximeter

Do google search about the aforementioned Pulse Oximeters for Continuous Monitoring, and purchase one of them for home use. The sales person or the technical team of the manufacturer of the pulse oximeter would train you over the phone on how to use the unit, and how to upload the data to your computer early in the morning after completing the test overnight, and how to generate a report on your computer, and how to understand the report.

III. DO YOUR OWN OVERNIGHT PULSE OXIMETRY TEST AT HOME CONFIDENTLY

<u>Take control of your health into your own hands</u>. Do not depend on hospitals, doctors, nurses, or CPAP vendors who can do the "overnight pulse oximetry test" for you. Do your own test, and learn how to do it confidently on your own if you want to reverse or improve your sleep apnea.

The sales person or the technical team of the manufacturer of the pulse oximeter would train you over the phone on how to use the unit, and how to upload the data to your computer early in the morning after completing the test overnight, and how to generate a report on your computer, and how to understand the report.

IV. LEARN HOW TO USE THE CPAP MACHINE CONFIDENTLY
DO NOT USE FULL-FACE MASK UNLESS YOU ARE ACCUSTOMED TO IT
FULL-FACE MASK CAN BE ANNOYING TO MANY PEOPLE

Best (Top 5) CPAP Machines of 2020, Recommended by CPAP.Com:
1. ResMed AirSense 10 AutoSet
2. ResMed AirMini AutoSet
3. Philips Respironics DreamStation Auto
4. Philips Respironics DreamStation Go
5. Z2 Auto Travel CPAP Machine

Understand how the CPAP machine works and find out a mask that is most comfortable. The following CPAP machine and mask were found to be the most comfortable and easy-to-use by the author of this book:
a. ResMed AirSense 10 Autoset CPAP Machine [36]
b. Philips Respironics Nuance Pro Gel Nasal Pillow Mask [39]

◉ Do some research within your community or city before you purchase the CPAP. Purchase the CPAP only from a reliable and trustworthy company. Most CPAP vendors offer 30-day free trial for using the CPAP. So you can use the 30-day free trial of several companies and finally select a machine that is most reliable and makes you feel comfortable. Make sure that the vendor offers free "overnight pulse oximetry test" with a continuous pulse oximeter once every few months. When you purchase the CPAP machine, make sure it comes with 30-day money back guarantee and 1-year warranty. Start using the CPAP therapy as soon as you are diagnosed with obstructive sleep apnea. <u>The CPAP therapy is the best therapy to control sleep apnea</u>.

◉ Research showed that "the average use of CPAP among sleep apnea patients is only 4-5 hours per night, not the recommended 7 1/2 hours a night." Many sleep apnea patients do not tolerate the CPAP machine and noisy mask, and so remove it in the middle of the night, and sleep without it the rest of the night. This kind of habit would lead to adverse and deadly consequences.

◉ In order to receive the successful therapy, a sleep apnea patient must use the CPAP therapy at least 7 hour a day. To be always on the safe side, if you have moderate or severe sleep apnea, you must not sleep even an hour without CPAP. When a sleep apnea patient sleeps without CPAP, his/her SpO2 level drops to a dangerous level below normal, suffocate himself or herself, and contributes to heart disease, sudden heart attack, and even death.

◉ **CPAP means "Continuous Positive Airway Pressure,"** which further means that the CPAP machine helps maintain continuous, positive, very low and comfortable pressure in the airway of your throat, keeps the airway open all the time, and stops snoring whenever you sleep with it. The CPAP machine has a mini compressor in it, which blows air into the mouth and/or nose at a very low and comfortable pressure, and keeps the airway always open by preventing the soft tissue of the throat muscles from collapsing onto the airway, thereby unblocking, abolishing snoring, shallow breathing and oxygen desaturation events. As long as you wear the CPAP machine during the night while sleeping, the CPAP machine kills most apneas and hypopneas, and keeps your AHI (Apnea Hypopnea Index) perfectly normal, under 5. As the airway remains always open, sufficient amount of air passes into the lungs freely, and maintains normal blood oxygen level (SpO2 = 96% to 99%) all the time during sleep. You wake up in the morning fully satisfied with your sleep and completely refreshed. You would not experience any symptoms of obstructive sleep apnea such as tiredness, low energy or lack of breath when you wake up in the morning.

◉ As you sleep all the night with perfectly normal SpO2 levels, your overall health improves. If you take appropriate steps to lose your excess body weight, your obstructive sleep apnea will be progressively healed and even reversed.

V. WIDE FLUCTUATIONS OF THE SpO2 LEVEL ARE DANGEROUS
FLATTEN THESE WIDE FLUCTUATIONS AND LET THEM STABILIZE

Watch the following Youtube videos in which Mr. James explains the SpO2 versus Time chart. You can see wide fluctuations in the SPO2 levels, which is dangerous when a person with obstructive sleep apnea sleeps. For example, when your blood oxygen level (SpO2) goes down significantly, your heart rate spikes. You should not only lower your SpO2 level to normal, but also minimize wide fluctuations in the SpO2 levels. You can accomplish this by sleeping with the CPAP machine continuously every night for at least 8 hours per night for 6 months to one year.

This Youtube Video Explains The Pulse Oximeter and SpO2 Versus Time Chart by James.
https://www.youtube.com/watch?v=cv3bfT8KqFc   (Pulse Oximeter)
https://www.youtube.com/watch?v=LiNi5hFGzrQ   (SpO2 Chart)
This Video Explains the SpO2 Versus Time Chart.
http://www.sleep-apnea-guide.com/sleep-apnea-oxygen-level.html

VI. LEARN HOW TO CALCULATE YOUR EXCESS BODY WEIGHT

For the complete weight-loss course, refer to another book titled REVERSING OBESITY (Self-Discovered Weight-Loss Method Illustrated) by Dr. RK who reversed his obstructive sleep apnea by losing weight. www.reversingsleepapnea.com/ebook2.html

a. Body Mass Index (BMI)

If you are diagnosed with obstructive sleep apnea, check how much excess weight you have. You can figure that out by calculating your current body mass index (BMI) and the excess body weight you have. You should lose weight until your Body Mass Index (BMI) drops to normal.

$$BMI = Weight (Kg) / [Height (m)]^2$$

Table 11.2 Assessment guidelines for BMI.

BMI (Kg/m^2)	Assessment
< 18.5	Underweight
18.5 to 24.9	Normal
25.0 to 29.9	Overweight
≥ 30	Obese

- Find out your weight in Kg (1 Kg = 2.2222 lb).
- Find out your height in meters.
 1 Foot = 0.3048 Meter; 1 Inch = 0.0254 Meters; 1 Meter = 3.281; 1 Feet = 39.37 inches

AN EXAMPLE CALCULATION OF BMI

Suppose Your Weight = 86 Kg, Your Height = 1.68 Meters
Your BMI = $(86)/(1.68)^2$ = 30.5 = That means you are "Obese".

HOW TO CALCULATE THE EXCESS BODY WEIGHT?

Body Mass Index (BMI) is calculated in metric units as follows:
$$BMI = Weight (Kg) / [Height (m)]^2$$

- If the weight is known in pounds, convert to Kg.
- If the height is known in feet and inches, convert to meters.
- Substitute the values in the formula, and then calculate the BMI.

Conversion Factors
1 Kg = 2.2222 Pounds; 1 Pound = 0.45 Kg
1 Meter = 3.281 Feet = 39.37 Inches
1 Foot = 0.3048 Meter, 1 Inch = 0.0254 Meter

Sample Calculation of BMI

George is 5' 6" tall and currently weighs 190 pounds (lb).
How many pounds should George lose to lower his body mass index (BMI) to normal?
Height = 5' 6" = 66 Inches = (66)(0.0254) = 1.6764 m
Weight = 190 lb = (190/2.2222) = 85.50 Kg
BMI = $(85.50)/(1.6764)^2$ = 30.42   Assessment = Obese

Sample Calculation of Excess Body Weight

a. Find out your weight in Kg (1 Kg = 2.2222 lb).
b. Find out your height in meters (1 meter = 3.281 feet = 39.37 inches).
c. For a normal BMI of less than or equal to 24.9, what would be your weight?
d. Calculate your normal weight (Kg) by substituting the values in the formula.
e. By knowing your current weight (Kg), and your normal weight that you just calculated, find out the excess body weight you have.

For a healthy weight, let us suppose reasonably that the BMI should be equal to or less than 24.5. So George's goal should be to lower his BMI from 30.29 to 24.5.

Using the aforementioned formula for BMI, the weight that corresponds to a BMI of 24.5 is calculated as follows:

$$BMI = \text{Weight (Kg)} / [\text{Height (m)}]^2$$
$$24.5 = \text{Weight (Kg)} / [1.68]^2$$
$$\text{Therefore Weight (Kg)} = (24.5)[1.68]^2$$
$$= (24.5)(1.68)(1.68)$$
$$= 68.85 \text{ Kg (which is the normal weight)}$$

Excess Body Weight of George = 85.50 – 68.85 = 16.65 Kg = 36.99 lb

That means George should lose at least 16.65 Kg or 37 pounds to lower his Body Mass Index (BMI) to normal.

IF YOU DON'T LIKE CALCULATIONS

If you have any difficulty of doing calculations or if you don't like calculations at all, then use the following website of National Heart, Lung and Blood Institute to find out your body mass index (BMI):
https://www.nhlbi.nih.gov/health/educational/lose_wt/BMI/bmicalc.htm
You simply enter your weight (pounds) and height (feet, inches) , it will calculate BMI for you.

b. Body Fat Percentage Using Omron Body Fat Analyzer

If the body mass index (BMI) formula does not suit your body type, check your body fat percentage using a body-fat analyzer. This kind of device is available in some pharmacies for free. You can go to a pharmacy, and monitor your body fat percentage every week. You should lose weight until your body fat percentage drops to normal. Your body fat percentage should be under 25%.

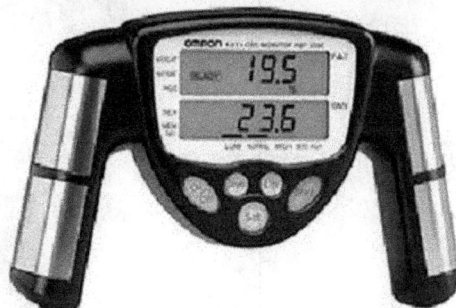

Courtesy of Omron Corp.
Figure 11.1 Omron body fat analyzer.

c. Body Fat Percentage Using Calipers Technique

You can also determine your body fat percentage by using this method. In some local gyms and community centers, some personal trainers are trained to perform the "body fat percentage using Calipers" by simply taking some measurements of the person's body. They will then calculate the body fat percentage from some simple formulae. You should lose weight until your body fat percentage drops to normal. Your body fat percentage should be under 25%.

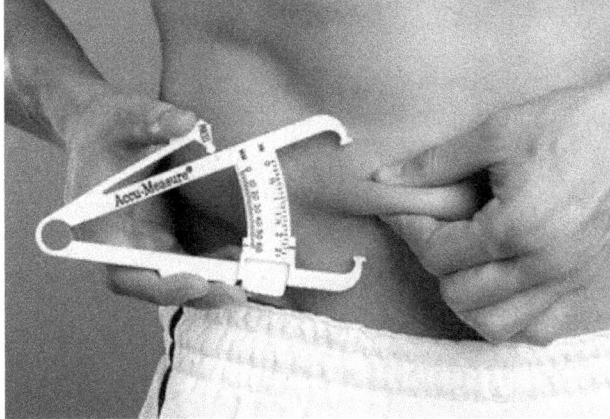

Figure 11.2 Body fat percentage using calipers technique.

d. Waist Circumference

The measurement of waist circumference is another indicative of body fat. When you have excess body fat and thus excess body weight, your waist circumference grows to an unacceptable level. In such cases, you must take immediate action to lower your waist circumference to normal. Each adult person has his/her own normal waist ranging from 30 inches to 34 inches, depending on the height of the person.

If your Body Mass Index (BMI) is normal or if your body fat percentage is normal, your waist would automatically look normal. If you have excess body weight or excess body fat, your waist would automatically look abnormal.

According to the US National Institutes of Health (NIH), a waist circumference in excess of 40 inches (or 102 centimeters) for men and a waist circumstance in excess of 35 inches (88 centimeters) for women poses high risk, and could cause type 2 diabetes, dyslipidemia, high blood pressure and several other health concerns.

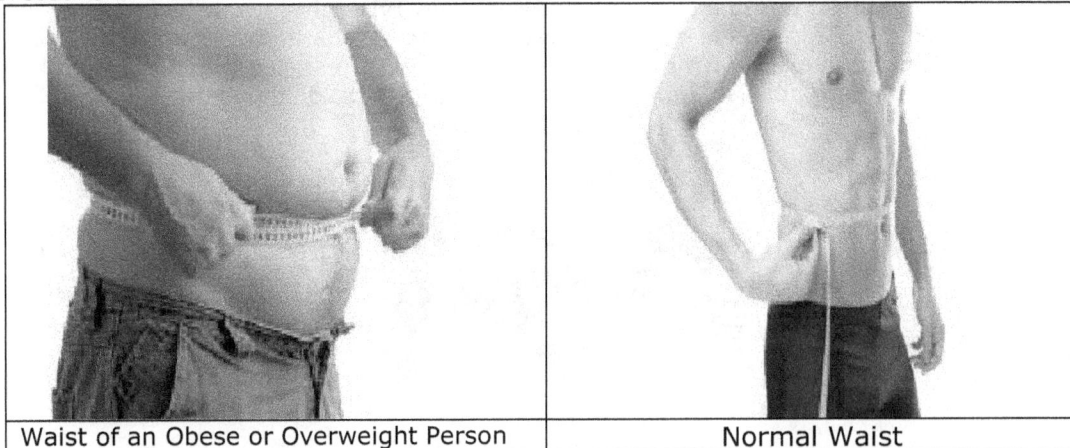

| Waist of an Obese or Overweight Person | Normal Waist |

Figure 11.3 Waist circumference of obese person and normal person.

VII. LEARN HOW TO LOSE ALL YOUR EXCESS BODY WEIGHT

Do your own research on "How to Lose Weight?" and develop a method to lose weight that suits your body, your situation, and your interests. And learn how to lose all that excess body weight.

VIII. WEIGHT LOSS RECOMMENDATIONS

It Is the most important commitment to be made if you want to reverse obstructive sleep apnea. The following recommendations might help you.

Create a 2000-Calorie Diet (low fat, high protein) with organic whole foods only.

- Learn how to recognize whole foods, processed foods and refined foods. Eliminate processed foods & refined foods from your diet. Eat only whole foods. Stop eating out in restaurants. Start eating at home meals made from whole foods.
- Learn how to count calories (if it is difficult for you, use measuring cups).
- Learn how to read labels when you shop for groceries. Eliminate foods with preservatives, artificial colors & flavors, saturated fat, trans fat, MSG, etc.
- Drink 8 to 16 cups of purified water every day. Extreme weight loss contestants drink 16 cups of water per day.
- Take apple cider vinegar (2 to 3 tbsp) in a cup of water using a STRAW before meals. It acts as a hunger suppressant, improves digestion and promotes weight loss.
- Eat organic Kamut Puffs as a snack whenever you feel hungry in between meals.
- Eat an omelet made with organic egg whites & veggies as a pre-workout meal.
- Exercise every day for an hour after eating the pre-workout meal.
- Minimize the salt and oil consumption in all your meals.
- Sleep at least 8 hours a night with the CPAP. If you have insomnia, fix it first.
- Record your weight and waist size every day when you wake up in the morning.
- Record your BMI once every week, making every effort to lower it to normal (< 25 Kg/m^2).

Go on with the 2000-Calorie Diet along with daily exercise for 2 to 3 months.
If you do not lose significant amount of weight, then lower the daily calorie intake by 500 calories and continue for another 2 or 3 months. For example,

a. After 3 months, create a new diet by reducing 2000 calories to 1500 calories.
b. After 3 more months, create a new diet by reducing 1500 calories to 1000 calories.
c. After 3 more months, create a new diet by reducing 1000 calories to 600 calories.

IMPORTANT NOTE: Please do not try a diet below 600 calories per day.

For the complete weight-loss course, refer to another book titled REVERSING OBESITY: Self-Discovered Weight-Loss Method Illustrated by Dr. RK who reversed his obesity and obstructive sleep apnea simultaneously simply by losing weight. Please visit
www.reversingsleepapnea.com/ebook2.html   (Reversing Obesity)
www.reversingsleepapnea.com   (Reversing Sleep Apnea)

AUTHOR'S NOTE: Did You Know? When I reduced my daily calorie intake from 2000 calories to 1000 calories, and stopped eating all junk foods (processed foods and refined foods), and maintained high willpower and high self-discipline, my body fat (mostly belly fat) melted away day by day right in front of my eyes, and I lost weight quickly. When my body resumed normal weight, my obstructive sleep apnea automatically disappeared. My Desaturation Index stunningly dropped from 28 events/hr to 0.6 Event/hr (less than 1 event per hour) in 22 months. I am now free from obstructive sleep apnea. I no longer sleep with the CPAP machine.

IX. THE MOST IMPORTANT RECOMMENDATION
FURTHER GUIDANCE

● Even some 10 to 20 pounds of weight loss would have a significant impact on your obstructive sleep apnea progress. The number of sleep apnea events per hour, what is known as Desaturation Index, during your sleep would significantly decline and the wide fluctuations of SpO2 would stabilize, switching you from severe sleep apnea to moderate sleep apnea, or from moderate sleep apnea to mild sleep apnea, and allowing you to feel a lot better than you have ever felt since your diagnosis.

● You don't have to fully or perfectly reverse your obstructive sleep apnea! If you could manage to switch your Desaturation Index from severe to moderate, or from moderate to mild, that would still be a great accomplishment. Try it out and improve your Desaturation Index (Number of sleep apnea events per hour during the sleep), you will feel a lot better and your overall health improves!

● With determination and steadfastness, you can not only improve your condition or sleep disorder, but also strengthen your ability to respond to your body's functionality and lead a much better life. You should always remember that knowledge is the power, so you must equip your mind with a deep understanding of sleep apnea by collecting as much information as possible, and by reading and researching a lot. Get ready to lower your Desaturation Index and the wide fluctuations of SpO2 during the sleep.

● Your biggest decision is your commitment to setting goals and objectives, focusing on your goal and staying focused until you fully manifest your goal. Motivation, commitment, a strong desire to succeed, self-discipline and high willpower are the essential qualities you need to implement on yourself to be successful. By awakening the giant within yourself, you can become a sleep apnea guru.

BEST WISHES!

About the Author

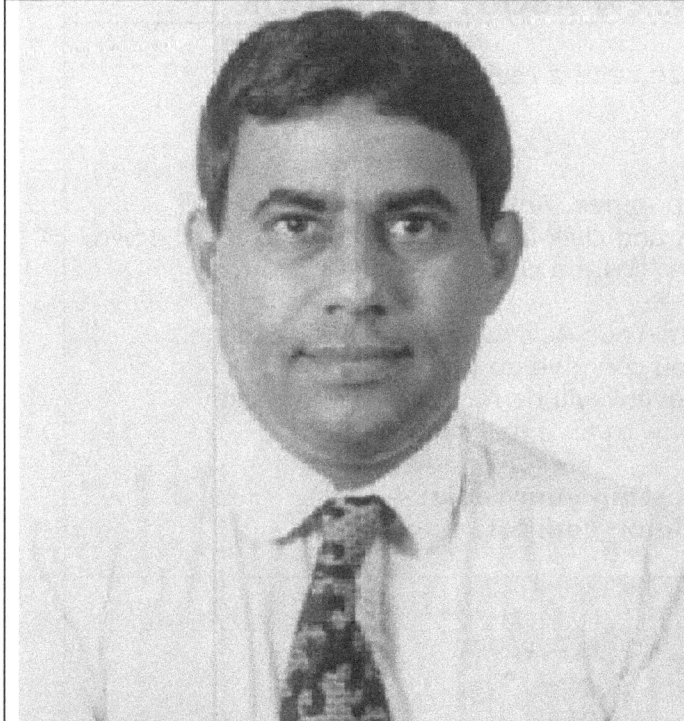

Dr. Rao M Konduru was a Chemical Engineer, and held two Master's degrees and two doctorates and two post-doctoral titles, all in chemical engineering. He published a book in 2003 titled "Permanent Diabetes Control," which earned immense respect and appreciation. Many people said it was a wonderful book. After suffering from a sudden heart attack in 1998, even though his left artery was 75% clogged with severe angina, he said "NO" to bypass surgery. He did what none of us would even think of doing. He simply relied on his natural self-prevention diet and exercise, and with it he reversed his critical diabetic heart disease in a matter of months, and developed a method to accomplish Permanent Diabetes Control. He also came up with a trial-and-error procedure to determine the optimal insulin dose that would tightly control diabetes, and would allow a diabetic person to live like a normal person for the rest of his/her life.

Dr. Rao M Konduru maintained his hemoglobin A1c level under 6.0% consistently. His personal best hemoglobin A1c level of 5.0% was an extraordinary result any diabetic person would hope to accomplish in a lifetime. Perhaps Dr. Rao M Konduru was the only diabetic person lived in this world with "Permanent Diabetes Control".

Once again, health demons such as uncontrollable weight gain, sleep apnea and chronic insomnia came his way. He did not give up, but persisted on discovering new, natural and effortless treatments of his own in reversing these most difficult disorders. His extensive scientific research experience and his powerful knowledge helped him battle and combat these life challenges. He figured out their root causes, and developed natural yet powerful techniques to cure these health disorders himself. After losing 40 pounds of weight and 12 inches around the waist, he successfully reversed his obesity, obstructive sleep apnea and chronic insomnia. He carefully created and published the following excellent guidebooks on Amazon so that others can benefit and be inspired to achieve similar results. His most recent book "Drinking Water Guide" is a 540-page book of wealth of information on drinking water for the rest of us.

1. Permanent Diabetes Control   www.mydiabetescontrol.com
2. The Secret to Controlling Type 2 Diabetes   www.mydiabetescontrol.com
3. Reversing Obesity   www.reversingsleepapnea.com/ebook2.html
4. Reversing Sleep Apnea   www.reversingsleepapnea.com
5. Reversing Insomnia   www.reversinginsomnia.com
6. Reversing Insomnia in 3 Days   www.reversinginsomnia.com
7. Drinking Water Guide   www.drinkingwaterguide.com
8. Drinking Water Guide-II   www.drinkingwaterguide.com
9. The Origin of the Earth's Water   www.drinkingwaterguide.com
10. Autobiography Of Dr. Rao M Konduru   www.mydiabetescontrol.com/Bio/

- Prime Publishing Co.

PLEASE WRITE A REVIEW ABOUT THIS BOOK

Now that you have read this book, please write a review about this book, and post your review on Amazon.

a. Please log into your Amazon account,
b. Search for this book "Reversing Sleep Apnea, Author: Rao Konduru, PhD", or by using ISBN # 9780973112023, and click on the book cover & scroll down,
c. Click on "Customer Reviews", click on "Write a customer review" button, and "Create Review" box pops up.
d. Kindly write your REVIEW in the Write-Your-Review box, type a Headline, and click on 5 stars overall rating (you can give up to 5 stars).
e. Click on "Submit" button, and your review will be registered on Amazon.
f. Amazon will acknowledge your review with an email confirmation!

Thanks for posting your review!
Your opinion counts!

YOUR OPINION COUNTS!

Kindle eBook Is Available on Amazon

You can read this book on your computer, laptop, tablet, e-reader, iPhone, or any Kindle device by purchasing Kindle eBook. It is available on Amazon.
Please log into your Amazon account, and search for "Reversing Sleep Apnea, Kindle eBook" or by using ASIN # B07L2347F9.

The end of the book "Reversing Sleep Apnea".

BEST WISHES!